The Works of Simone de Beauvoir

by Simone de Beauvoir

Includes:

The Ethics of Ambiguity, 1947

The Second Sex, 1949

On the publication of The Second Sex, 1963 interview

Biography

Printed in the U.S.A.

2011

The Works of Simone de Beauvoir

Table of Contents

The Second Sex

Introduction
Woman as Other

FOR a long time I have hesitated to write a book on woman. The subject is irritating, especially to women; and it is not new. Enough ink has been spilled in quarrelling over feminism, and perhaps we should say no more about it. It is still talked about, however, for the voluminous nonsense uttered during the last century seems to have done little to illuminate the problem. After all, is there a problem? And if so, what is it? Are there women, really? Most assuredly the theory of the eternal feminine still has its adherents who will whisper in your ear: 'Even in Russia women still are women'; and other erudite persons – sometimes the very same – say with a sigh: 'Woman is losing her way, woman is lost.' One wonders if women still exist, if they will always exist, whether or not it is desirable that they should, what place they occupy in this world, what their place should be. 'What has become of women?' was asked recently in an ephemeral magazine.

But first we must ask: what is a woman? 'Tota mulier in utero', says one, 'woman is a womb'. But in speaking of certain women, connoisseurs declare that they are not women, although they are equipped with a uterus like the rest. All agree in recognising the fact that females exist in the human species; today as always they make up about one half of humanity. And yet we are told that femininity is in danger; we are exhorted to be women, remain women, become women. It would appear, then, that every female human being is not necessarily a woman; to be so considered she must share in that mysterious and threatened reality known as femininity. Is this attribute something secreted by the ovaries? Or is it a Platonic essence, a product of the philosophic imagination? Is a rustling petticoat enough to bring it down to earth? Although some women try zealously to incarnate this essence, it is hardly patentable. It is frequently described in vague and dazzling terms that seem to have been borrowed from the vocabulary of the seers, and indeed in the times of St Thomas it was considered an essence as certainly defined as the somniferous virtue of the poppy

But conceptualism has lost ground. The biological and social sciences no longer admit the existence of unchangeably fixed entities that determine given characteristics, such as those ascribed to woman, the Jew, or the Negro. Science regards any characteristic as a reaction dependent in part upon a *situation*. If today femininity no longer exists, then it never existed. But does the word *woman*, then, have no specific content? This is stoutly affirmed by those who hold to the philosophy of the enlightenment, of rationalism, of nominalism; women, to them, are merely the human beings arbitrarily designated by the word *woman*. Many American women particularly are prepared to think that there is no longer any place for woman as such; if a backward individual still takes herself for a woman, her friends advise her to be psychoanalysed and thus get rid of this obsession. In regard to a work, *Modern Woman: The Lost Sex*, which in other respects has its irritating features, Dorothy Parker has written: 'I cannot be just to books which treat of woman as woman ... My idea is that all of us, men as well as women, should be regarded as human beings.' But nominalism is a rather inadequate doctrine, and the antifeminists have had no trouble in showing that women simply *are* not men. Surely woman is, like man, a human being; but such a declaration is abstract. The fact is that every concrete human being is always a singular, separate individual. To decline to accept such notions as the eternal feminine, the black soul, the Jewish character, is not to deny that Jews, Negroes, women exist today – this denial does not represent a liberation for those concerned, but rather a flight from reality. Some years ago a well-known woman writer refused to permit her portrait to appear in a series of photographs especially devoted to women writers; she wished to be counted among the men. But in order to gain this privilege she made use of her husband's influence! Women who assert that they are men lay claim none the less to masculine consideration and respect. I recall also a young Trotskyite standing on a platform at a boisterous meeting and getting ready to use her fists, in spite of her evident fragility. She was denying her feminine weakness; but it was for love of a militant male whose equal she wished to be. The attitude of defiance of many American women proves that they are haunted by a sense of their femininity. In truth, to go for a walk with one's eyes open is enough to demonstrate that humanity is divided into two classes of individuals whose clothes, faces, bodies, smiles, gaits, interests, and occupations are manifestly different. Perhaps these differences are superficial, perhaps they are destined to disappear. What is certain is that they do most obviously exist.

If her functioning as a female is not enough to define woman, if we decline also to explain her through 'the eternal feminine', and if nevertheless we admit, provisionally, that women do exist, then we must face the question "what is a woman"?

To state the question is, to me, to suggest, at once, a preliminary answer. The fact that I ask it is in itself significant. A man would never set out to write a book on the peculiar situation of the human male. But if I wish to define myself, I must first of all say: 'I am a woman'; on this truth must be based all further discussion. A man never begins by presenting himself as an individual of a certain sex; it goes without saying that he is a man. The terms *masculine* and *feminine* are used symmetrically only as a matter of form, as on legal papers. In actuality the relation of the two sexes is not quite like that of two electrical poles, for man represents both the positive and the neutral, as is indicated by the common use of *man* to designate human beings in general; whereas woman represents only the negative, defined by limiting criteria, without reciprocity. In the midst of an abstract discussion it is vexing to hear a man say: 'You think thus and so because you are a woman'; but I know that my only defence is to reply: 'I think thus and so because it is true,' thereby removing my subjective self from the argument. It would be out of the question to reply: 'And you think the contrary because you are a man', for it is understood that the fact of being a man is no peculiarity. A man is in the right in being a man; it is the woman who is in the wrong. It amounts to this: just as for the ancients there was an absolute vertical with reference to which the oblique was defined, so there is an absolute human type, the masculine. Woman has ovaries, a uterus: these peculiarities imprison her in her subjectivity, circumscribe her within the limits of her own nature. It is often said that she thinks with her glands. Man superbly ignores the fact that his anatomy also includes glands, such as the testicles, and that they secrete hormones. He thinks of his body as a direct and normal connection with the world, which he believes he apprehends objectively, whereas he regards the body of woman as a hindrance, a prison, weighed down by everything peculiar to it. 'The female is a female by virtue of a certain lack of qualities,' said Aristotle; 'we should regard the female nature as afflicted with a natural defectiveness.' And St Thomas for his part pronounced woman to be an 'imperfect man', an 'incidental' being. This is symbolised in Genesis where Eve is depicted as made from what Bossuet called 'a supernumerary bone' of Adam.

Thus humanity is male and man defines woman not in herself but as relative to him; she is not regarded as an autonomous being. Michelet writes: 'Woman, the relative being ...' And Benda is most positive in his *Rapport d'Uriel*: 'The body of man makes sense in itself quite apart from that of woman, whereas the latter seems wanting in significance by itself ... Man can think of himself without woman. She cannot think of herself without man.' And she is simply what man decrees; thus she is called 'the sex', by which is meant that she appears essentially to the male as a sexual being. For him she is sex – absolute sex, no less. She is defined and differentiated with reference to man and not he with reference to her; she is the incidental, the inessential as opposed to the essential. He is the Subject, he is the Absolute – she is the Other.'

The category of the *Other* is as primordial as consciousness itself. In the most primitive societies, in the most ancient mythologies, one finds the expression of a duality – that of the Self and the Other. This duality was not originally attached to the division of the sexes; it was not dependent upon any empirical facts. It is revealed in such works as that of Granet on Chinese thought and those of Dumézil on the East Indies and Rome. The feminine element was at first no more involved in such pairs as Varuna-Mitra, Uranus-Zeus, Sun-Moon, and Day-Night than it was in the contrasts between Good and Evil, lucky and unlucky auspices, right and left, God and Lucifer. Otherness is a fundamental category of human thought.

Thus it is that no group ever sets itself up as the One without at once setting up the Other over against itself. If three travellers chance to occupy the same compartment, that is enough to make vaguely hostile 'others' out of all the rest of the passengers on the train.

In small-town eyes all persons not belonging to the village are 'strangers' and suspect; to the native of a country all who inhabit other countries are 'foreigners'; Jews are 'different' for the anti-Semite, Negroes are 'inferior' for American racists, aborigines are 'natives' for colonists, proletarians are the 'lower class' for the privileged.

Lévi-Strauss, at the end of a profound work on the various forms of primitive societies, reaches the following conclusion: 'Passage from the state of Nature to the state of Culture is marked by man's ability to view biological relations as a series of contrasts; duality, alternation, opposition, and symmetry, whether under definite or vague forms, constitute not so much phenomena to be explained as fundamental and immediately given data of social reality.' These phenomena would be incomprehensible if in fact human society were simply a *Mitsein* or fellowship based on solidarity and friendliness. Things become clear, on the contrary, if, following Hegel, we find in consciousness itself a fundamental hostility towards every other consciousness; the subject can be posed only in being opposed – he sets himself up as the essential, as opposed to the other, the inessential, the object.

But the other consciousness, the other ego, sets up a reciprocal claim. The native travelling abroad is shocked to find himself in turn regarded as a 'stranger' by the natives of neighbouring countries. As a matter of fact, wars, festivals, trading, treaties, and contests among tribes, nations, and classes tend to deprive the concept *Other* of its absolute sense and to make manifest its relativity; willy-nilly, individuals and groups are forced to realize the reciprocity of their relations. How is it, then, that this reciprocity has not been recognised between the sexes, that one of the contrasting terms is set up as the sole essential, denying any relativity in regard to its correlative and defining the latter as pure otherness? Why is it that women do not dispute male sovereignty? No subject will readily volunteer to become the object, the inessential; it is not the Other who, in defining himself as the Other, establishes the One. The Other is posed as such by the One in defining himself as the One. But if the Other is not to regain the status of being the One, he must be submissive enough to accept this alien point of view. Whence comes this submission in the case of woman?

There are, to be sure, other cases in which a certain category has been able to dominate another completely for a time. Very often this privilege depends upon inequality of numbers – the majority imposes its rule upon the minority or persecutes it. But women are not a minority, like the American Negroes or the Jews; there are as many women as men on earth. Again, the two groups concerned have often been originally independent; they may have been formerly unaware of each other's existence, or perhaps they recognised each other's autonomy. But a historical event has resulted in the subjugation of the weaker by the stronger. The scattering of the Jews, the introduction of slavery into America, the conquests of imperialism are examples in point. In these cases the oppressed retained at least the memory of former days; they possessed in common a past, a tradition, sometimes a religion or a culture.

The parallel drawn by Bebel between women and the proletariat is valid in that neither ever formed a minority or a separate collective unit of mankind. And instead of a single historical event it is in both cases a historical development that explains their status as a class and accounts for the membership of *particular individuals* in that class. But proletarians have not always existed, whereas there have always been women. They are women in virtue of their anatomy and physiology. Throughout history they have always been subordinated to men, and hence their dependency is not the result of a historical event or a social change – it was not something that *occurred*. The reason why otherness in this case seems to be an absolute is in part that it lacks the contingent or incidental nature of historical facts. A condition brought about at a certain time can be abolished at some other time, as the Negroes of Haiti and others have proved: but it might seem that natural condition is beyond the possibility of change. In truth, however, the nature of things is no more immutably given, once for all, than is historical reality. If woman seems to be the inessential which never becomes the essential, it is because she herself fails to bring about this change. Proletarians say 'We'; Negroes also. Regarding themselves as subjects, they transform the bourgeois, the whites, into 'others'. But women do not say 'We', except at some congress of feminists or similar formal demonstration; men say 'women', and women use the same word in referring to themselves. They do not authentically assume a subjective attitude. The proletarians have accomplished the revolution in Russia, the Negroes in Haiti, the Indo-Chinese are battling for it in Indo-China; but the women's effort has never been anything more than a symbolic agitation. They have gained only what men have been willing to grant; they have taken nothing, they have only received.

The reason for this is that women lack concrete means for organising themselves into a unit which can stand face to face with the correlative unit. They have no past, no history, no religion of their own; and they have no such solidarity of work and interest as that of the proletariat. They are not even promiscuously herded together in the way that creates community feeling among the American Negroes, the ghetto Jews, the workers of Saint-Denis, or the factory hands of Renault. They live dispersed among the males, attached through residence, housework, economic condition, and social standing to certain men – fathers or husbands – more firmly than they are to other women. If they belong to the bourgeoisie, they feel solidarity with men of that class, not with proletarian women; if they are white, their allegiance is to white men, not to Negro women. The proletariat can propose to massacre the ruling class, and a sufficiently fanatical Jew or Negro might dream of getting sole possession of the atomic bomb and making humanity wholly Jewish or black; but woman cannot even dream of exterminating the males. The bond that unites her to her oppressors is not comparable to any other. The division of the sexes is a biological fact, not an event in human history. Male and female stand opposed within a primordial *Mitsein*, and woman has not broken it. The couple is a fundamental unity with its two halves riveted together, and the cleavage of society along the line of sex is impossible. Here is to be found the basic trait of woman: she is the Other in a totality of which the two components are necessary to one another.

One could suppose that this reciprocity might have facilitated the liberation of woman. When Hercules sat at the feet of Omphale and helped with her spinning, his desire for her held him captive; but why did she fail to gain a lasting power? To revenge herself on Jason, Medea killed their children; and this grim legend would seem to suggest that she might have obtained a formidable influence over him through his love for his offspring. In *Lysistrata* Aristophanes gaily depicts a band of women who joined forces to gain social ends through the sexual needs of their men; but this is only a play. In the legend of the Sabine women, the latter soon abandoned their plan of remaining sterile to punish their ravishers. In truth woman has not been socially emancipated through man's need – sexual desire and the desire for offspring – which makes the male dependent for satisfaction upon the female.

Master and slave, also, are united by a reciprocal need, in this case economic, which does not liberate the slave. In the relation of master to slave the master does not make a point of the need that he has for the other; he has in his grasp the power of satisfying this need through his own action; whereas the slave, in his dependent condition, his hope and fear, is quite conscious of the need he has for his master. Even if the need is at bottom equally urgent for both, it always works in favour of the oppressor and against the oppressed. That is why the liberation of the working class, for example, has been slow.

Now, woman has always been man's dependant, if not his slave; the two sexes have never shared the world in equality. And even today woman is heavily handicapped, though her situation is beginning to change. Almost nowhere is her legal status the same as man's, and frequently it is much to her disadvantage. Even when her rights are legally recognised in the abstract, long-standing custom prevents their full expression in the mores. In the economic sphere men and women can almost be said to make up two castes; other things being equal, the former hold the better jobs, get higher wages, and have more opportunity for success than their new competitors. In industry and politics men have a great many more positions and they monopolise the most important posts. In addition to all this, they enjoy a traditional prestige that the education of children tends in every way to support, for the present enshrines the past – and in the past all history has been made by men. At the present time, when women are beginning to take part in the affairs of the world, it is still a world that belongs to men – they have no doubt of it at all and women have scarcely any. To decline to be the Other, to refuse to be a party to the deal – this would be for women to renounce all the advantages conferred upon them by their alliance with the superior caste. Man-the-sovereign will provide woman-the-liege with material protection and will undertake the moral justification of her existence; thus she can evade at once both economic risk and the metaphysical risk of a liberty in which ends and aims must be contrived without assistance. Indeed, along with the ethical urge of each individual to affirm his subjective existence, there is also the temptation to forgo liberty and become a thing. This is an inauspicious road, for he who takes it – passive, lost, ruined – becomes henceforth the creature of another's will, frustrated in his transcendence and deprived of every value. But it is an easy road; on it one avoids the strain involved in undertaking an authentic existence. When man makes of woman the Other, he may, then, expect to manifest deep-seated tendencies towards complicity. Thus, woman may fail to lay claim to the status of subject because she lacks definite resources, because she feels the necessary bond that ties her to man regardless of reciprocity, and because she is often very well pleased with her role as the Other.

But it will be asked at once: how did all this begin? It is easy to see that the duality of the sexes, like any duality, gives rise to conflict. And doubtless the winner will assume the status of absolute. But why should man have won from the start? It seems possible that women could have won the victory; or that the outcome of the conflict might never have been decided. How is it that this world has always belonged to the men and that things have begun to change only recently? Is this change a good thing? Will it bring about an equal sharing of the world between men and women?

These questions are not new, and they have often been answered. But the very fact that woman *is the Other* tends to cast suspicion upon all the justifications that men have ever been able to provide for it. These have all too evidently been dictated by men's interest. A little-known feminist of the seventeenth century, Poulain de la Barre, put it this way: 'All that has been written about women by men should be suspect, for the men are at once judge and party to the lawsuit.' Everywhere, at all times, the males have displayed their satisfaction in feeling that they are the lords of creation. 'Blessed be God ... that He did not make me a woman,' say the Jews in their morning prayers, while their wives pray on a note of resignation: 'Blessed be the Lord, who created me according to His will.' The first among the blessings for which Plato thanked the gods was that he had been created free, not enslaved; the second, a man, not a woman. But the males could not enjoy this privilege fully unless they believed it to be founded on the absolute and the eternal; they sought to make the fact of their supremacy into a right. 'Being men, those who have made and compiled the laws have favoured their own sex, and jurists have elevated these laws into principles', to quote Poulain de la Barre once more.

Legislators, priests, philosophers, writers, and scientists have striven to show that the subordinate position of woman is willed in heaven and advantageous on earth. The religions invented by men reflect this wish for domination. In the legends of Eve and

Pandora men have taken up arms against women. They have made use of philosophy and theology, as the quotations from Aristotle and St Thomas have shown. Since ancient times satirists and moralists have delighted in showing up the weaknesses of women. We are familiar with the savage indictments hurled against women throughout French literature. Montherlant, for example, follows the tradition of Jean de Meung, though with less gusto. This hostility may at times be well founded, often it is gratuitous; but in truth it more or less successfully conceals a desire for self-justification. As Montaigne says, 'It is easier to accuse one sex than to excuse the other'. Sometimes what is going on is clear enough. For instance, the Roman law limiting the rights of woman cited 'the imbecility, the instability of the sex' just when the weakening of family ties seemed to threaten the interests of male heirs. And in the effort to keep the married woman under guardianship, appeal was made in the sixteenth century to the authority of St Augustine, who declared that 'woman is a creature neither decisive nor constant', at a time when the single woman was thought capable of managing her property. Montaigne understood clearly how arbitrary and unjust was woman's appointed lot: 'Women are not in the wrong when they decline to accept the rules laid down for them, since the men make these rules without consulting them. No wonder intrigue and strife abound.' But he did not go so far as to champion their cause.

It was only later, in the eighteenth century, that genuinely democratic men began to view the matter objectively. Diderot, among others, strove to show that woman is, like man, a human being. Later John Stuart Mill came fervently to her defence. But these philosophers displayed unusual impartiality. In the nineteenth century the feminist quarrel became again a quarrel of partisans. One of the consequences of the industrial revolution was the entrance of women into productive labour, and it was just here that the claims of the feminists emerged from the realm of theory and acquired an economic basis, while their opponents became the more aggressive. Although landed property lost power to some extent, the bourgeoisie clung to the old morality that found the guarantee of private property in the solidity of the family. Woman was ordered back into the home the more harshly as her emancipation became a real menace. Even within the working class the men endeavoured to restrain woman's liberation, because they began to see the women as dangerous competitors – the more so because they were accustomed to work for lower wages.

In proving woman's inferiority, the anti-feminists then began to draw not only upon religion, philosophy, and theology, as before, but also upon science – biology, experimental psychology, etc. At most they were willing to grant 'equality in difference' to the other sex. That profitable formula is most significant; it is precisely like the 'equal but separate' formula of the Jim Crow laws aimed at the North American Negroes. As is well known, this so-called equalitarian segregation has resulted only in the most extreme discrimination. The similarity just noted is in no way due to chance, for whether it is a race, a caste, a class, or a sex that is reduced to a position of inferiority, the methods of justification are the same. 'The eternal feminine' corresponds to 'the black soul' and to 'the Jewish character'. True, the Jewish problem is on the whole very different from the other two – to the anti-Semite the Jew is not so much an inferior as he is an enemy for whom there is to be granted no place on earth, for whom annihilation is the fate desired. But there are deep similarities between the situation of woman and that of the Negro. Both are being emancipated today from a like paternalism, and the former master class wishes to 'keep them in their place' – that is, the place chosen for them. In both cases the former masters lavish more or less sincere eulogies, either on the virtues of 'the good Negro' with his dormant, childish, merry soul – the submissive Negro – or on the merits of the woman who is 'truly feminine' – that is, frivolous, infantile, irresponsible the submissive woman. In both cases the dominant class bases its argument on a state of affairs that it has itself created. As George Bernard Shaw puts it, in substance, 'The American white relegates the black to the rank of shoeshine boy; and he concludes from this that the black is good for nothing but shining shoes.' This vicious circle is met with in all analogous circumstances; when an individual (or a group of individuals) is kept in a situation of inferiority, the fact is that he is inferior. But the significance of the verb *to be* must be rightly understood here; it is in bad faith to give it a static value when it really has the dynamic Hegelian sense of 'to have become'. Yes, women on the whole ***are*** today inferior to men; that is, their situation affords them fewer possibilities. The question is: should that state of affairs continue?

Many men hope that it will continue; not all have given up the battle. The conservative bourgeoisie still see in the emancipation of women a menace to their morality and their interests. Some men dread feminine competition. Recently a male student wrote in the *Hebdo-Latin*: 'Every woman student who goes into medicine or law robs us of a job.' He never questioned his rights in this world. And economic interests are not the only ones concerned. One of the benefits that oppression confers upon the oppressors is that the most humble among them is made to feel superior; thus, a 'poor white' in the South can console himself with the thought that he is not a 'dirty nigger' – and the more prosperous whites cleverly exploit this pride.

Similarly, the most mediocre of males feels himself a demigod as compared with women. It was much easier for M. de Montherlant to think himself a hero when he faced women (and women chosen for his purpose) than when he was obliged to act the man among men – something many women have done better than he, for that matter. And in September 1948, in one of his articles in the *Figaro littéraire*, Claude Mauriac – whose great originality is admired by all – could write regarding woman: 'We listen on a tone [*sic!*] of polite indifference ... to the most brilliant among them, well knowing that her wit reflects more or less luminously ideas that come from *us*.' Evidently the speaker referred to is not reflecting the ideas of Mauriac himself, for no one knows of his having any. It may be that she reflects ideas originating with men, but then, even among men there are those who have been known to appropriate ideas not their own; and one can well ask whether Claude Mauriac might not find more interesting a conversation reflecting Descartes, Marx, or Gide rather than himself. What is really remarkable is that by using the questionable *we* he identifies himself with St Paul, Hegel, Lenin, and Nietzsche, and from the lofty eminence of their grandeur looks down disdainfully upon the bevy of women who make bold to converse with him on a footing of equality. In truth, I know of more than one woman who would refuse to suffer with patience Mauriac's 'tone of polite indifference'.

I have lingered on this example because the masculine attitude is here displayed with disarming ingenuousness. But men profit in many more subtle ways from the otherness, the alterity of woman. Here is a miraculous balm for those afflicted with an inferiority complex, and indeed no one is more arrogant towards women, more aggressive or scornful, than the man who is anxious about his virility. Those who are not fear-ridden in the presence of their fellow men are much more disposed to recognise a fellow creature in woman; but even to these the myth of Woman, the Other, is precious for many reasons. They cannot be blamed for not cheerfully relinquishing all the benefits they derive from the myth, for they realize what they would lose in relinquishing woman as they fancy her to be, while they fail to realize what they have to gain from the woman of tomorrow. Refusal to pose oneself as the Subject, unique and absolute, requires great self-denial. Furthermore, the vast majority of men make no such claim explicitly. They do not *postulate* woman as inferior, for today they are too thoroughly imbued with the ideal of democracy not to recognise all human beings as equals.

In the bosom of the family, woman seems in the eyes of childhood and youth to be clothed in the same social dignity as the adult males. Later on, the young man, desiring and loving, experiences the resistance, the independence of the woman desired and loved; in marriage, he respects woman as wife and mother, and in the concrete events of conjugal life she stands there before him as a free being. He can therefore feel that social subordination as between the sexes no longer exists and that on the whole, in spite of differences, woman is an equal. As, however, he observes some points of inferiority – the most important being unfitness for the professions – he attributes these to natural causes. When he is in a co-operative and benevolent relation with woman, his theme is the principle of abstract equality, and he does not base his attitude upon such inequality as may exist. But when he is in conflict with her, the situation is reversed: his theme will be the existing inequality, and he will even take it as justification for denying abstract equality.

So it is that many men will affirm as if in good faith that women are the equals of man and that they have nothing to clamour for, while *at the same time* they will say that women can never be the equals of man and that their demands are in vain. It is, in point of fact, a difficult matter for man to realize the extreme importance of social discriminations which seem outwardly insignificant but which produce in woman moral and intellectual effects so profound that they appear to spring from her original nature. The most sympathetic of men never fully comprehend woman's concrete situation. And there is no reason to put much trust in the men when they rush to the defence of privileges whose full extent they can hardly measure. We shall not, then, permit ourselves to be intimidated by the number and violence of the attacks launched against women, nor to be entrapped by the self-seeking eulogies bestowed on the 'true woman', nor to profit by the enthusiasm for woman's destiny manifested by men who would not for the world have any part of it.

We should consider the arguments of the feminists with no less suspicion, however, for very often their controversial aim deprives them of all real value. If the 'woman question' seems trivial, it is because masculine arrogance has made of it a 'quarrel'; and when quarrelling one no longer reasons well. People have tirelessly sought to prove that woman is superior, inferior, or equal to man. Some say that, having been created after Adam, she is evidently a secondary being: others say on the contrary that Adam was only a rough draft and that God succeeded in producing the human being in perfection when He created Eve. Woman's brain is smaller; yes, but it is relatively larger. Christ was made a man; yes, but perhaps for his greater humility. Each argument at once suggests its opposite, and both are often fallacious. If we are to gain understanding, we must get out of these ruts; we must discard the vague notions of superiority, inferiority, equality which have hitherto corrupted every discussion of the subject and start afresh.

Very well, but just how shall we pose the question? And, to begin with, who are we to propound it at all? Man is at once judge and party to the case; but so is woman. What we need is an angel – neither man nor woman – but where shall we find one? Still, the angel would be poorly qualified to speak, for an angel is ignorant of all the basic facts involved in the problem. With a hermaphrodite we should be no better off, for here the situation is most peculiar; the hermaphrodite is not really the combination of a whole man and a whole woman, but consists of parts of each and thus is neither. It looks to me as if there are, after all, certain women who are best qualified to elucidate the situation of woman. Let us not be misled by the sophism that because Epimenides was a Cretan he was necessarily a liar; it is not a mysterious essence that compels men and women to act in good or in bad faith, it is their situation that inclines them more or less towards the search for truth. Many of today's women, fortunate in the restoration of all the privileges pertaining to the estate of the human being, can afford the luxury of impartiality – we even recognise its necessity. We are no longer like our partisan elders; by and large we have won the game. In recent debates on the status of women the United Nations has persistently maintained that the equality of the sexes is now becoming a reality, and already some of us have never had to sense in our femininity an inconvenience or an obstacle. Many problems appear to us to be more pressing than those which concern us in particular, and this detachment even allows us to hope that our attitude will be objective. Still, we know the feminine world more intimately than do the men because we have our roots in it, we grasp more immediately than do men what it means to a human being to be feminine; and we are more concerned with such knowledge. I have said that there are more pressing problems, but this does not prevent us from seeing some importance in asking how the fact of being women will affect our lives. What opportunities precisely have been given us and what withheld? What fate awaits our younger sisters, and what directions should they take? It is significant that books by women on women are in general animated in our day less by a wish to demand our rights than by an effort towards clarity and understanding. As we emerge from an era of excessive controversy, this book is offered as one attempt among others to confirm that statement.

But it is doubtless impossible to approach any human problem with a mind free from bias. The way in which questions are put, the points of view assumed, presuppose a relativity of interest; all characteristics imply values, and every objective description, so called, implies an ethical background. Rather than attempt to conceal principles more or less definitely implied, it is better to state them openly, at the beginning. This will make it unnecessary to specify on every page in just what sense one uses such words as *superior, inferior, better, worse, progress, reaction*, and the like. If we survey some of the works on woman, we note that one of the points of view most frequently adopted is that of the public good, the general interest; and one always means by this the benefit of society as one wishes it to be maintained or established. For our part, we hold that the only public good is that which assures the private good of the citizens; we shall pass judgement on institutions according to their effectiveness in giving concrete opportunities to individuals. But we do not confuse the idea of private interest with that of happiness, although that is another common point of view. Are not women of the harem more happy than women voters? Is not the housekeeper happier than the working-woman? It is not too clear just what the word *happy* really means and still less what true values it may mask. There is no possibility of measuring the happiness of others, and it is always easy to describe as happy the situation in which one wishes to place them.

In particular those who are condemned to stagnation are often pronounced happy on the pretext that happiness consists in being at rest. This notion we reject, for our perspective is that of existentialist ethics. Every subject plays his part as such specifically through exploits or projects that serve as a mode of transcendence; he achieves liberty only through a continual reaching out towards other liberties. There is no justification for present existence other than its expansion into an indefinitely open future. Every time transcendence falls back into immanence, stagnation, there is a degradation of existence into the '*en-sois*' – the brutish life of subjection to given conditions – and of liberty into constraint and contingence. This downfall represents a moral fault if the subject consents to it; if it is inflicted upon him, it spells frustration and oppression. In both cases it is an absolute evil. Every individual concerned to justify his existence feels that his existence involves an undefined need to transcend himself, to engage in freely chosen projects.

Now, what peculiarly signalises the situation of woman is that she – a free and autonomous being like all human creatures – nevertheless finds herself living in a world where men compel her to assume the status of the Other. They propose to stabilise her as object and to doom her to immanence since her transcendence is to be overshadowed and for ever transcended by another ego (*conscience*) which is essential and sovereign. The drama of woman lies in this conflict between the fundamental aspirations of every subject (ego) – who always regards the self as the essential and the compulsions of a situation in which she is the inessential. How can a human being in woman's situation attain fulfilment? What roads are open to her? Which are blocked? How can independence be recovered in a state of dependency? What circumstances limit woman's liberty and how can they be overcome? These are the fundamental questions on which I would fain throw some light. This means that I am interested in the fortunes of the individual as defined not in terms of happiness but in terms of liberty.

Quite evidently this problem would be without significance if we were to believe that woman's destiny is inevitably determined by physiological, psychological, or economic forces. Hence I shall discuss first of all the light in which woman is viewed by biology, psychoanalysis, and historical materialism. Next I shall try to show exactly how the concept of the 'truly feminine' has been fashioned – why woman has been defined as the Other – and what have been the consequences from man's point of view. Then from woman's point of view I shall describe the world in which women must live; and thus we shall be able to envisage the difficulties in their way as, endeavouring to make their escape from the sphere hitherto assigned them, they aspire to full membership in the human race.

The Second Sex
by Simone de Beauvoir (1949)

Book One: Facts and Myths, Part I: Destiny

Chapter 1, The Data of Biology

WOMAN? Very simple, say the fanciers of simple formulas: she is a womb, an ovary; she is a female – this word is sufficient to define her. In the mouth of a man the epithet female has the sound of an insult, yet he is not ashamed of his animal nature; on the contrary, he is proud if someone says of him: 'He is a male!' The term 'female' is derogatory not because it emphasises woman's animality, but because it imprisons her in her sex; and if this sex seems to man to be contemptible and inimical even in harmless dumb animals, it is evidently because of the uneasy hostility stirred up in him by woman. Nevertheless he wishes to find in biology a justification for this sentiment. The word *female* brings up in his mind a saraband of imagery – a vast, round ovum engulfs and castrates the agile spermatozoan; the monstrous and swollen termite queen rules over the enslaved males; the female praying mantis and the spider, satiated with love, crush and devour their partners; the bitch in heat runs through the alleys, trailing behind her a wake of depraved odours; the she-monkey presents posterior immodestly and then steals away with hypocritical coquetry; and the most superb wild beasts – the tigress, the lioness, the panther – bed down slavishly under the imperial embrace of the male. Females sluggish, eager, artful, stupid, callous, lustful, ferocious, abased – man projects them all at once upon woman. And the fact is that she is a female. But if we are willing to stop thinking in platitudes, two questions are immediately posed: what does the female denote in the animal kingdom? And what particular kind of female is manifest in woman?

Males and females are two types of individuals which are differentiated within a species for the function of reproduction; they can be defined only correlatively. But first it must be noted that even the division of a species into two sexes is not always clear-cut.

In nature it is not universally manifested. To speak only of animals, it is well known that among the microscopic one-celled forms – infusoria, amoebae, sporozoans, and the like – multiplication is fundamentally distinct from sexuality. Each cell divides and subdivides by itself. In many-celled animals or metazoans reproduction may take place asexually, either by schizogenesis – that is, by fission or cutting into two or more parts which become new individuals – or by blastogenesis – that is, by buds that separate and form new individuals. The phenomena of budding observed in the fresh-water hydra and other coelenterates, in sponges, worms, and tunicates, are well-known examples. In cases of parthenogenesis the egg of the virgin female develops into an embryo without fertilisation by the male, which thus may play no role at all. In the honey-bee copulation takes place, but the eggs may or may not be fertilised at the time of laying. The unfertilised eggs undergo development and produce the drones (males); in the aphids males are absent during a series of generations in which the eggs are unfertilised and produce females. Parthenogenesis has been induced artificially in the sea urchin, the starfish, the frog, and other species. Among the one-celled animals (Protozoa), however, two cells may fuse, forming what is called a zygote; and in the honey-bee fertilisation is necessary if the eggs are to produce females. In the aphids both males and females appear in the autumn, and the fertilised eggs then produced are adapted for over-wintering.

Certain biologists in the past concluded from these facts that even in species capable of asexual propagation occasional fertilisation is necessary to renew the vigour of the race –

to accomplish 'rejuvenation' through the mixing of hereditary material from two individuals. On this hypothesis sexuality might well appear to be an indispensable function in the most complex forms of life; only the lower organisms could multiply without sexuality, and even here vitality would after a time become exhausted. But today this hypothesis is largely abandoned; research has proved that under suitable conditions asexual multiplication can go on indefinitely without noticeable degeneration, a fact that is especially striking in the bacteria and Protozoa. More and more numerous and daring experiments in parthenogenesis are being performed, and in many species the male appears to be fundamentally unnecessary. Besides, if the value of intercellular exchange were demonstrated, that value would seem to stand as a sheer, unexplained fact. Biology certainly demonstrates the existence of sexual differentiation, but from the point of view of any end to be attained the science could not infer such differentiation from the structure of the cell, nor from the laws of cellular multiplication, nor from any basic phenomenon.

The production of two types of gametes, the sperm and the egg, does not necessarily imply the existence of two distinct sexes; as a matter of fact, egg and sperm – two highly differentiated types of reproductive cells – may both be produced by the same individual. This occurs in normally hermaphroditic species, which are common among plants and are also to be found among the lower animals, such as annelid worms and molluscs. In them reproduction may be accomplished through self-fertilisation or, more commonly, cross-fertilisation. Here again certain biologists have attempted to account for the existing state of affairs. Some hold that the separation of the gonads (ovaries and testes) in two distinct individuals represents an evolutionary advance over hermaphroditism; others on the contrary regard the separate condition as primitive, and believe that hermaphroditism represents a degenerate state. These notions regarding the superiority of one system or the other imply the most debatable evolutionary theorising. All that we can say for sure is that these two modes of reproduction coexist in nature, that they both succeed in accomplishing the survival of the species concerned, and that the differentiation of the gametes, like that of the organisms producing them, appears to be accidental. It would seem, then, that the division of a species into male and female individuals is simply an irreducible fact of observation.

In most philosophies this fact has been taken for granted without pretence of explanation. According to the Platonic myth, there were at the beginning men, women, and hermaphrodites. Each individual had two faces, four arms, four legs, and two conjoined bodies. At a certain time they were split in two, and ever since each half seeks to rejoin its corresponding half. Later the gods decreed that new human beings should be created through the coupling of dissimilar halves. But it is only love that this story is intended to explain; division into sexes is assumed at the outset. Nor does Aristotle explain this division, for if matter and form must cooperate in all action, there is no necessity for the active and passive principles to he separated in two different categories of individuals. Thus St Thomas proclaims woman an 'incidental' being, which is a way of suggesting – from the male point of view – the accidental or contingent nature of sexuality. Hegel, however, would have been untrue to his passion for rationalism had he failed to attempt a logical explanation. Sexuality in his view represents the medium through which the subject attains a concrete sense of belonging to a particular kind (genre). 'The sense of kind is produced in the subject as an effect which offsets this disproportionate sense of his individual reality, as a desire to find the sense of himself in another individual of his species through union with this other, to complete himself and thus to incorporate the kind (genre) within his own nature and bring it into existence. This is copulation' (*Philosophy of Nature*, Part 3, Section 369). And a little farther on. 'The process consists in this, namely: that which they are in themselves, that is to say a single kind, one and the same subjective life, they also establish it as such.' And Hegel states later that for the uniting process to be accomplished, there must first be sexual differentiation. But his exposition is not convincing: one feels in it all too distinctly the predetermination to find in every operation the three terms of the syllogism.

The projection or transcendence of the individual towards the species, in which both individual and species are fulfilled, could be accomplished without the intervention of a third element in the simple relation of progenitor to offspring; that is to say, reproduction could be asexual. Or, if there were to be two progenitors, they could be similar (as happens in hermaphroditic species) and differentiated only as particular individuals of a single type. Hegel's discussion reveals a most important significance of sexuality, but his mistake is always to argue from significance to necessity, to equate significance with necessity. Man gives significance to the sexes and their relations through sexual activity, just as he gives sense and value to all the functions that he exercises; but sexual activity is not necessarily implied in the nature of the human being. Merleau-Ponty notes in the *Phénoménologie de la perception* that human existence requires us to revise our ideas of necessity and contingence. 'Existence,' he says, 'has no casual, fortuitous qualities, no content that does not contribute to the formation of its aspect; it does not admit the notion of sheer fact, for it is only through existence that the facts are manifested.' True enough. But it is also true that there are conditions without which the very fact of existence itself would seem to be impossible. To be present in the world implies strictly that there exists a body which is at once a material thing in the world and a point of view towards this world; but nothing requires that this body have this or that particular structure. Sartre discusses in *L'Étre et le néant* Heidegger's dictum to the effect that the real nature of man is bound up with death because of man's finite state. He shows that an existence which is finite and yet unlimited in time is conceivable; but none the less if death were not resident in human life, the relation of man to the world and to himself would be profoundly disarranged – so much so that the statement 'Man is mortal' would be seen to have significance quite other than that of a mere fact of observation. Were he immortal, an existent would no longer be what we call a man. One of the essential features of his career is that the progress of his life through time creates behind him and before him the infinite past and future, and it would seem, then, that the perpetuation of the species is the correlative of his individual limitation. Thus we can regard the phenomenon of reproduction as founded in the very nature of being. But we must stop there. The perpetuation of the species does not necessitate sexual differentiation. True enough, this differentiation is characteristic of existents to such an extent that it belongs in any realistic definition of existence. But it nevertheless remains true that both a mind without a body and an immortal man are strictly inconceivable, whereas we can imagine a parthenogenetic or hermaphroditic society.

On the respective functions of the two sexes man has entertained a great variety of beliefs. At first they had no scientific basis, simply reflecting social myths. It was long thought – and it still is believed in certain primitive matriarchal societies – that the father plays no part in conception. Ancestral spirits in the form of living germs are supposed to find their way into the maternal body. With the advent patriarchal institutions, the male laid eager claim to his posterity. It was still necessary to grant the mother a part in procreation, but it was conceded only that she carried and nourished the living seed, created by the father alone. Aristotle fancied that the foetus arose from the union of sperm and menstrual blood, woman furnishing only passive matter while the male principle contributed force, activity, movement, life. Hippocrates held to a similar doctrine, recognising two kinds of seed, the weak or female and the strong or male. The theory of Aristotle survived through the Middle Ages and into modern times.

At the end of the seventeenth century Harvey killed female dogs shortly after copulation and found in the horns of the uterus small sacs that he thought were eggs but that were really embryos. The Danish anatomist Steno gave the name of ovaries to the female genital glands, previously called 'feminine testicles', and noted on their surface the small swellings that von Graaf in 1677 erroneously identified with the eggs and that are now called Graafian follicles. The ovary was still regarded as homologous to the male gland. In the same year, however, the 'spermatic animalcules' were discovered and it was proved that they penetrated into the uterus of the female; but it was supposed that they were simply nourished therein and that the coming individual was preformed in them. In 1694 a Dutchman, Hartsaker, drew a picture of the 'homunculus' hidden in the spermatozoan, and in 1699, another scientist said that he had seen the spermatozoan cast off a kind of moult under which appeared a little man, which he also drew. Under these imaginative hypotheses, woman was restricted to the nourishment of an active, living principle already preformed in perfection. These notions were not universally accepted, and they were argued into the nineteenth century. The use of the microscope enabled von Baer in 1827 to discover the mammalian egg, contained inside the Graaflan follicle. Before long it was possible to study the cleavage of the egg – that is, the early stage of development through cell division – and in 1835 sarcode, later called protoplasm, was discovered and the true nature of the cell began to be realised. In 1879 the penetration of the spermatozoan into the starfish egg was observed, and thereupon the equivalence of the nuclei of the two gametes, egg and sperm, was established. The details of their union within the fertilised egg were first worked out in 1883 by a Belgian zoologist, van Beneden.

Aristotle's ideas were not wholly discredited, however. Hegel held that the two sexes were of necessity different, the one active and the other passive, and of course the female would be the passive one. 'Thus man, in consequence of that differentiation, is the active principle while woman is the passive principle because she remains undeveloped in her unity.' [Hegel, *Philosophy of Nature*] And even after the egg had been recognised as an active principle, men still tried to make a point of its quiescence as contrasted with the lively movements of the sperm. Today one notes an opposite tendency on the part of some scientists. The discoveries made in the course of experiments on parthenogenesis have led them to reduce the function of the sperm to that of a simple physico-chemical reagent. It has been shown that in certain species the stimulus of an acid or even of a needle-prick is enough to initiate the cleavage of the egg and the development of the embryo. On this basis it has been boldly suggested that the male gamete (sperm) is not necessary for reproduction, that it acts at most as a ferment; further, that perhaps in time the co-operation of the male will become unnecessary in procreation – the answer, it would seem, to many a woman's prayer. But there is no warrant for so bold an expectation, for nothing warrants us in universalising specific life processes. The phenomena of asexual propagation and of parthenogenesis appear to be neither more nor less fundamental than those of sexual reproduction. I have said that the latter has no claim *a priori* to be considered basic; but neither does any fact indicate that it is reducible to any more fundamental mechanism.

Thus, admitting no *a priori* doctrine, no dubious theory, we are confronted by a fact for which we can offer no basis in the nature of things nor any explanation through observed data, and the significance of which we cannot comprehend *a priori*. We can hope to grasp the significance of sexuality only by studying it in its concrete manifestations; and then perhaps the meaning of the word female will stand revealed.

I do not intend to offer here a philosophy of life; and I do not care to take sides prematurely in the dispute between the mechanistic and the purposive or teleological philosophies. It is to be noted, however, that all physiologists and biologists use more or less finalistic language, if only because they ascribe meaning to vital phenomena. I shall adopt their terminology without taking any stand on the relation between life and consciousness, we can assert that every biological fact implies transcendence, that every function involves a project, something to be done. Let my words be taken to imply no more than that.

In the vast majority of species male and female individuals co-operate in reproduction. They are defined primarily as male and female by the gametes which they produce – sperms and eggs respectively. In some lower plants and animals the cells that fuse to form the zygote are identical; and these cases of isogamy are significant because they illustrate the basic equivalence of the gametes. In general the gametes are differentiated, and yet their equivalence remains a striking fact. Sperms and eggs develop from similar primordial germ cells in the two sexes. The development of oocytes from the primordial cells in the female differs from that of spermatocytes in the male chiefly in regard to the protoplasm, but the nuclear phenomena are clearly the same. The biologist Ancel suggested in 1903 that the primordial germ cell is indifferent and undergoes development into sperm or egg depending upon which type of gonad, testis or ovary, contains it. However this may be, the primordial germ cells of each sex contain the same number of chromosomes (that characteristic of the species concerned), which number is reduced to one half by closely analogous processes in male and female. At the end of these developmental processes (called spermatogenesis in the male and oogenesis in the female) the gametes appear fully matured as sperms and eggs, differing enormously in some respects, as noted below, but being alike in that each contains a single set of equivalent chromosomes.

Today it is well known that the sex of offspring is determined by the chromosome constitution established at the time of fertilisation. According to the species concerned, it is either the male gamete or the female gamete that accomplishes this result. In the mammals it is the sperm, of which two kinds are produced in equal numbers, one kind containing an X-chromosome (as do all the eggs), the other kind containing a Y-chromosome (not found in the eggs). Aside from the X- and Y-chromosomes, egg and sperm contain an equivalent set of these bodies. It is obvious that when sperm and egg unite in fertilisation, 'the fertilised egg will contain two full sets of chromosomes, making up the number characteristic of the species – 48 in man, for example. If fertilisation is accomplished by an X-bearing sperm, the fertilised egg will contain two X-chromosomes and will develop into a female (XX). If the Y-bearing sperm fertilises the egg, only one X-chromosome will be present and the sex will be male (XY). In birds and butterflies the situation is reversed, though the principle remains the same; it is the eggs that contain either X or Y and hence determine the sex the offspring. In the matter of heredity, the laws of Mendel show 'that the father and the mother play equal parts. The chromosomes contain the factors of heredity (genes), and they are conveyed equally in egg and sperm.

What we should note in particular at this point is that neither gamete can be regarded as superior to the other; when they unite, both lose their individuality in the fertilised egg. There are two common suppositions which – at least on this basic biological level – are clearly false. The first – that of the passivity of the female – is disproved by the fact that new life springs from the union of the two gametes; the living spark is not the exclusive property of either. The nucleus of the egg is a centre of vital activity exactly symmetrical with the nucleus of the sperm. The second false supposition contradicts the first – which does not seem to prevent their coexistence. It is to the effect that the permanence of the species is assured by the female, the principle being of an explosive and transitory nature. As a matter of fact, the embryo carries on the germ plasm of the father as well as that of the mother and transmits them together to its descendants under now male, now female form. It is, so to speak, an androgynous germ plasm, which outlives the male or female individuals that are its incarnations, whenever they produce offspring.

This said, we can turn our attention to secondary differences between egg and sperm, which are of the greatest interest. The essential peculiarity of the egg is that it is provided with means for nourishing and protecting the embryo; it stores up reserve material from which the foetus will build its tissues, material that is not living substance but inert yolk. In consequence the egg is of massive, commonly spherical form and relatively large. The size of birds' eggs is well known; in woman the egg is almost microscopic, about equal in size to a printed period (diameter 0.132- 0.135 mm.), but the human sperm is far smaller (0.04 – 0.06 mm. in length), so small that a cubic millimetre would hold 60,000. The sperm has a threadlike tail and a small, flattened oval head, which contains the chromosomes. No inert substance weighs it down; it is wholly alive. In its whole structure it is adapted for mobility. Whereas the egg, big with the future of the embryo, is stationary; enclosed within the female body or floating externally in water, it passively awaits fertilisation. It is the male gamete that seeks it out. The sperm is always a naked cell; the egg may or may not be protected with shell and membranes according to the species; but in any case, when the sperm makes contact with the egg, it presses against it, sometimes shakes it, and bores into it. The tail is dropped and the head enlarges, forming the male nucleus, which now moves towards the egg nucleus. Meanwhile the egg quickly forms a membrane, which prevents the entrance of other sperms. In the starfish and other echinoderms, where fertilisation takes place externally, it is easy to observe the onslaught of the sperms, which surround the egg like an aureole. The competition involved is an important phenomenon, and it occurs in most species. Being much smaller than the egg, the sperm is generally produced in far greater numbers (more than 200,000,000 to 1 in the human species), and so each egg has numerous suitors.

Thus the egg – active in its essential feature, the nucleus – is superficially passive; its compact mass, sealed up within itself, evokes nocturnal darkness and inward repose. It was the form of the sphere that to the ancients represented the circumscribed world, the impenetrable atom. Motionless, the egg waits; in contrast the sperm – free, slender, agile – typifies the impatience and the restlessness of existence. But allegory should not be pushed too far. The ovule has sometimes been likened to immanence, the sperm to transcendence, and it has been said that the sperm penetrates the female element only in losing its transcendence, its motility; it is seized and castrated by the inert mass that engulfs it after depriving it of its tail. This is magical action – disquieting, as is all passive action – whereas the activity of the male gamete is rational; it is movement measurable in terms of time and space. The truth is that these notions are hardly more than vagaries of the mind. Male and female gametes fuse in the fertilised egg; they are both suppressed in becoming a new whole. It is false to say that the egg greedily swallows the sperm, and equally so to say that the sperm victoriously commandeers the female cell's reserves, since in the act of fusion the individuality of both is lost. No doubt movement seems to the mechanistic mind to be an eminently rational phenomenon, but it is an idea no clearer for modern physics than action at a distance. Besides, we do not know in detail the physico-chemical reactions that lead up to gametic union. We can derive a valid suggestion, however, from this comparison of the gametes. There are two interrelated dynamic aspects of life: it can be maintained only through transcending itself, and it can transcend itself only on condition that it is maintained. These two factors always operate together, and it is unrealistic to try to separate them, yet now it is one and now the other that dominates. The two gametes at once transcend and perpetuate themselves when they unite; but in its structure the egg anticipates future needs, it is so constituted as to nourish the life that will wake within it. The sperm, on the contrary, is in no way equipped to provide for the development of the embryo it awakens. On the other hand, the egg cannot provide the change of environment that will stimulate a new outburst of life, whereas the sperm can and does travel. Without the foresight of the egg, the sperm's arrival would be in vain; but without the initiative of the latter, the egg would not fulfil its living potentialities.

We may conclude, then, that the two gametes play a fundamentally identical role; together they create a living being in which both of them are at once lost and transcended. But in the secondary and superficial phenomena upon which fertilisation depends, it is the male element which provides the stimuli needed for evoking new life and it is the female element that enables this new life to be lodged in a stable organism.

It would be foolhardy indeed to deduce from such evidence that woman's place is in the home – but there are foolhardy men. In his book *Le Tempérament et le charactère*, Alfred Fouillée undertakes to found his definition of woman *in toto* upon the egg and that of man upon the spermatozoan; and a number of supposedly profound theories rest upon this play of doubtful analogies. It is a question to what philosophy of nature these dubious ideas pertain; not to the laws of heredity, certainly, for, according to these laws, men and women alike develop from an egg and a sperm. I can only suppose that in such misty minds there still float shreds of the old philosophy of the Middle Ages which taught that the cosmos is an exact reflection of a microcosm – the egg is imagined to be a little female, the woman a giant egg. These musings, generally abandoned since the days of alchemy, make a bizarre contrast with the scientific precision of the data upon which they are now based, for modern biology conforms with difficulty to medieval symbolism. But our theorisers do not look too closely into the matter. In all honesty it must be admitted that in any case it is a long way from the egg to woman. In the unfertilised egg not even the concept of femaleness is as yet established. As Hegel justly remarks the sexual relation cannot be referred back to the relation of the gametes. It is our duty, then, to study the female organism as a whole.

It has already been pointed out that in many plants and in some animals (such as snails) the presence of two kinds of gametes does not require two kinds of individuals, since every individual produces both eggs and sperms. Even when the sexes are separate, they are not distinguished in any such fashion as are different species. Males and females appear rather to be variations on a common groundwork, much as the two gametes are differentiated from similar original tissue. In certain animals (for example, the marine worm Bonellia) the larva is asexual, the adult becoming male or female according to the circumstances under which it has developed. But as noted above (pages 42-3), sex is determined in most species by the genotypic constitution of the fertilised egg. In bees the unfertilised eggs laid by the queen produce males exclusively; in aphids parthenogenetic eggs usually produce females. But in most animals all eggs that develop have been fertilised, and it is notable that the sexes are produced in approximately equal numbers through the mechanism of chromosomal sex-determination, already explained.

In the embryonic development of both sexes the tissue from which the gonads will be formed is at first indifferent; at a certain stage either testes or ovaries become established; and similarly in the development of the other sex organs there is an early indifferent period when the sex of the embryo cannot be told from an examination of these parts, from which, later on, the definitive male or female structures arise. All this helps to explain the existence of conditions intermediate between hermaphroditism and gonochorism (sexes separate). Very often one sex possesses certain organs characteristic of the other; a case in point is the toad, in which there is in the male a rudimentary ovary called Bidder's organ, capable of producing eggs under experimental conditions. Among the mammals there are indications of this sexual bipotentiality, such as the uterus masculinus and the rudimentary mammary glands in the male, and in the female Gärtner's canal and the clitoris. Even in those species exhibiting a high degree of sexual differentiation individuals combining both male and female characteristics may occur. Many cases of intersexuality are known in both animals and man; and among insects and crustaceans one occasionally finds examples of gynandromorphism, in which male and female areas of the body are mingled in a kind of mosaic.

The fact is that the individual, though its genotypic sex is fixed at fertilisation, can be profoundly affected by the environment in which it develops. In the ants, bees, and termites the larval nutrition determines whether the genotypic female individual will become a fully developed female ('queen') or a sexually retarded worker. In these cases the whole organism is affected; but the gonads do not play a part in establishing the sexual differences of the body, or soma. In the vertebrates, however, the hormones secreted by the gonads are the essential regulators. Numerous experiments show that by varying the hormonal (endocrine) situation, sex can be profoundly affected. Grafting and castration experiments on adult animals and man have contributed to the modern theory of sexuality, according to which the soma is in a way identical in male and female vertebrates. It may be regarded as a kind of neutral element upon which the influence of the gonad imposes the sexual characteristics. Some of the hormones secreted by the gonad act as stimulators, others as inhibitors. Even the genital tract itself is somatic, and embryological investigations show that it develops in the male or female direction from an indifferent and in some respects hermaphroditic condition under the hormonal influence. Intersexuality may result when the hormones are abnormal and hence neither one of the two sexual potentialities is exclusively realised.

Numerically equal in the species and developed similarly from like beginnings, the fully formed male and female are basically equivalent. Both have reproductive glands – ovaries or testes – in which the gametes are produced by strictly corresponding processes, as we have seen. These glands discharge their products through ducts that are more or less complex according to sex; in the female the egg may pass directly to the outside through the oviduct, or it may be retained for a time in the cloaca or the uterus before expulsion; in the male the semen may be deposited outside, or there may be a copulatory organ through which it is introduced into the body of the female. In these respects, then, male and female appear to stand in a symmetrical relation to each other. To reveal their peculiar, specific qualities it will be necessary to study them from the functional point of view.

It is extremely difficult to give a generally valid definition of the female. To define her as the bearer of the eggs and the male as bearer of the sperms is far from sufficient, since the relation of the organism to the gonads is, as we have seen, quite variable. On the other hand, the differences between the gametes have no direct effect upon the organism as a whole; it has sometimes been argued that the eggs, being large, consume more vital energy than do the sperms, but the latter are produced in such infinitely greater numbers that the expenditure of energy must be about equal in the two sexes. Some have wished to see in spermatogenesis an example of prodigality and in oogenesis a model of economy, but there is an absurd liberality in the latter, too, for the vast majority of eggs are never fertilised. In no way do gametes and gonads represent in microcosm the organism as a whole. It is to this the whole organism – that we must now direct our attention.

One of the most remarkable features to be noted as we survey the scale of animal life is that as we go up, individuality is seen to be more and more fully developed. At the bottom, life is concerned only in the survival of the species as a whole; at the top, life seeks expression through particular individuals, while accomplishing also the survival of the group. In some lower species the organism may be almost entirely reduced to the reproductive apparatus; in this case the egg, and hence the female, is supreme, since the egg is especially dedicated to the mere propagation of life; but here the female is hardly more than an abdomen, and her existence is entirely used up in a monstrous travail of ovulation. In comparison with the male, she reaches giant proportions; but her appendages are often tiny, her body a shapeless sac, her organs degenerated in favour of the eggs. Indeed, such males and females, although they are distinct organisms, can hardly be regarded as individuals, for they form a kind of unity made up of inseparable elements. In a way they are intermediate between hermaphroditism and gonochorism.

Thus in certain Crustacea, parasitic on the crab, the female is a mere sac enclosing millions of eggs, among which are found the minute males, both larval and adult. In *Edriolydnus* the dwarf male is still more degenerate; it lives under the shell of the female and has no digestive tract of its own, being purely reproductive in function. But in all such cases the female is no less restricted than the male; it is enslaved to the species. If the male is bound to the female, the latter is no less bound down, either to a living organism on which it exists as a parasite or to some substratum; and its substance is consumed in producing the eggs which the tiny male fertilises.

Among somewhat higher animals an individual autonomy begins to be manifested and the bond that joins the sexes weakens; but in the insects they both remain strictly subordinated to the eggs. Frequently, in the mayflies, male and female die immediately after copulation and egg-laying. In some rotifers the male lacks a digestive tract and fecundation; the female is able to eat and survives long least to develop and lay the eggs. The mother dies after the appearance of the next generation is assured. The privileged position held by the females in many insects comes from the fact that the production and sometimes the care of the eggs demand a long effort, whereas fecundation is for the most part quickly accomplished.

In the termites the enormous queen, crammed with nourishment and laying as many as 4,000 eggs per day until she becomes sterile and is pitilessly killed, is no less a slave than the comparatively tiny male who attends her and provides frequent fecundations. In the matriarchal ants' nests and beehives the males are economically useless and are killed off at times. At the season of the nuptial flight in ants, all the males emerge with females from the nest; those that succeed in mating with females die at once, exhausted; the rest are not permitted by the workers to re-enter the nest, and die of hunger or are killed. The fertilised female has a gloomy fate; she buries herself alone in the ground and often dies while laying her first eggs, or if she succeeds in founding a colony she remains shut in and may live for ten or twelve years constantly producing more eggs. The workers, females with atrophied sexuality, may live for several years, but their life is largely devoted to raising the larvae. It is much the same with bees; the drone that succeeds in mating with the queen during the nuptial flight falls to earth disembowelled; the other drones return to the hive, where they live a lazy life and are in the way until at the approach of winter they are killed off by the workers. But the workers purchase their right to live by incessant toil; as in the ants they are undeveloped females. The queen is in truth enslaved to the hive, laying eggs continually. If she dies, the workers give several larvae special food so as to provide for the succession; the first to emerge kills the rest in their cells.

In certain spiders the female carries the eggs about with her in a silken case until they hatch. She is much larger and stronger than the male and may kill and devour him after copulation, as does an insect, the praying mantis, around which has crystallised the myth of devouring femininity – the egg castrates the sperm, the mantis murders her spouse, these acts foreshadowing a feminine dream of castration. The mantis, however, shows her cruelty especially in captivity; and under natural conditions, when she is free in the midst of abundant food, she rarely dines on the male. If she does eat him, it is to enable her to produce her eggs and thus perpetuate the race, just as the solitary fertilised ant often eats some of her own eggs under the same necessity. It is going far afield to see in these facts a proclamation of the 'battle of the sexes' which sets individuals, as such, one against another. It cannot simply be said that in ants, bees, termites, spiders, or mantises the female enslaves and sometimes devours the male, for it is the species that in different ways consumes them both. The female lives longer and seems to be more important than the male; but she has no independence – egg-laying and the care of eggs and larvae are her destiny, other functions being atrophied wholly or in part.

In the male, on the contrary, an individual existence begins to be manifested. In impregnation he very often shows more initiative than the female, seeking her out, making the approach, palpating, seizing, and forcing connection upon her. Sometimes he has to battle for her with other males. Accordingly the organs of locomotion, touch, an prehension frequently more highly evolved in the male. Many female moths are wingless, while the males have wings; and often the males of insects have more highly developed colours, wing-covers, legs, and pincers. And sometimes to this endowment is added a seeming luxury of brilliant coloration. Beyond the brief moment of copulation the life of the male is useless and irresponsible; compared with the industriousness of the workers, the idleness of the drones seems a remarkable privilege. But this privilege is a social disgrace, and often the male pays with his life for his futility and partial independence. The species, which holds the female in slavery, punishes the male for his gesture towards escape; it liquidates him with brutal force.

In higher forms of life, reproduction becomes the creation of discrete organisms; it takes on a double role: maintenance of the species and creation of new individuals. This innovating aspect becomes the more unmistakable as the singularity of the individual becomes pronounced. It is striking that these, two essential elements – perpetuation and creation – are separately apportioned to the two sexes. This separation, already indicated at the moment when the egg is fertilised, is to be discerned in the whole generative process. It is not the essential nature of the egg that requires this separation, for in higher forms of life the female has, like the male, attained a certain autonomy and her bondage to the egg has been relaxed. The female fish, batrachian, or bird is far from being a mere abdomen. The less strictly the mother is bound to the egg, the less does the labour of reproduction represent an absorbing task and the more uncertainty there is in the relations of the two parents with their offspring. It can even happen that the father will take charge of the newly hatched young, as in various fishes.

Water is an element in which the eggs and sperms can float about and unite, and fecundation in the aquatic environment is almost always external. Most fish do not copulate, at most stimulating one another by contact. The mother discharges the eggs, the father the sperm – their role is identical. There is no reason why the mother, any more than the father, should feel responsibility for the eggs. In some species the eggs are abandoned by the parents and develop without assistance; sometimes a nest is prepared by the mother and sometimes she watches over the eggs after they have been fertilised. But very often it is the father who takes charge of them. As soon as he has fertilised them, he drives away the female to prevent her from eating them, and he protects them savagely against any intruder. Certain males have been described as making a kind of protective nest by blowing bubbles of air enclosed in an insulating substance; and in many cases they protect the developing eggs in their mouths or, as in the seahorse, in abdominal folds.

In the batrachians (frogs and toads) similar phenomena are to be seen. True copulation is unknown to them; they practise amplexus, the male embracing the female and thus stimulating her to lay her eggs. As the eggs are discharged, the sperms are deposited upon them. In the obstetrical toad the male wraps the strings of eggs about his hind legs and protects them, taking them into the water when the young are about to hatch as tadpoles.

In birds the egg is formed rather slowly inside the female; it is relatively large and is laid with some difficulty. It is much more closely associated with the mother than with the father, who has simply fertilised it in a brief copulation. Usually the mother sits on the eggs and takes care of the newly hatched young; but often the father helps in nest-building and in the protection and feeding of the young birds. In rare cases – for example among the sparrows – the male does the incubating and rearing. Male and female pigeons secrete in the crop a milky fluid with, which they both feed the fledglings. It is remarkable that in these cases where the male takes part in nourishing the young, there is no production of sperms during the time devoted to them while occupied in maintaining life the male has no urge to beget new living beings.

In the mammals life assumes the most complex forms, and individualisation is most advanced and specific. There the division of the two vital components – maintenance and creation – is realised definitively in the separation of the sexes. It is in this group that the mother sustains the closest relations – among vertebrates – with her offspring, and the father shows less interest in them. The female organism is wholly adapted for and subservient to maternity, while sexual initiative is the prerogative of the male.

The female is the victim of the species. During certain periods in the year, fixed in each species, her whole life is under the regulation of a sexual cycle (the oestrus cycle), of which the duration, as well as the rhythmic sequence of events, varies from one species to another. This cycle consists of two phases: during the first phase the eggs (variable in number according to the species) become mature and the lining of the uterus becomes thickened and vascular; during the second phase (if fertilisation has not occurred) the egg disappears, the uterine edifice breaks down, and the material is eliminated in a more or less noticeable temporary flow, known as menstruation in woman and related higher mammals. If fertilisation does occur, the second phase is replaced by pregnancy. The time of ovulation (at the end of the first phase) is known as oestrus and it corresponds to the period of rut, heat, or sexual activity.

In the female mammal, rut is largely passive; she is ready and waiting to receive the male. It may happen in mammals – as in certain birds – that she solicits the male, but she does no more than appeal to him by means of cries, displays, and suggestive attitudinising. She is quite unable to force copulation upon him. In the end it is he who makes the decision. We have seen that even in the insects, where the female is highly privileged in return for her total sacrifice to the species, it is usually the male who takes the initiative in fecundation; among the fishes he often stimulates the female to lay her eggs through his presence and contact; and in the frogs and toads he acts as a stimulator in amplexus. But it is in birds and mammals especially that he forces himself upon her, while very often she submits indifferently or even resists him.

Even when she is willing, or provocative, it is unquestionably the male who takes the female – she is taken. Often the word applies literally, for whether by means of special organs or through superior strength, the male seizes her and holds her in place; he performs the copulatory movements; and, among insects, birds, and mammals, he penetrates her. In this penetration her inwardness is violated, she is like an enclosure that is broken into. The male is not doing violence to the species, for the species survives only in being constantly renewed and would come to an end if eggs and sperms did not come together; but the female, entrusted with the protection of the egg, locks it away inside herself, and her body, in sheltering the egg, shields it also from the fecundating action of the male. Her body becomes, therefore, a resistance to be broken through, whereas in penetrating it the male finds self-fulfilment in activity.

His domination is expressed in the very posture of copulation – in almost all animals the male is on the female. And certainly the organ he uses is a material object, but it appears here in its animated state it is a tool – whereas in this performance the female organ is more in the nature of an inert receptacle. The male deposits his semen, the female receives it. Thus, though the female plays a fundamentally active role in procreation, she submits to the coition, which invades her individuality and introduces an alien element through penetration and internal fertilisation. Although she may feel the sexual urge as a personal need, since she seeks out the male when in heat, yet the sexual adventure is immediately experienced by her as an interior event and not as an outward relation to the world and to others.

But the fundamental difference between male and female mammals lies in this: the sperm, through which the life of the male is transcended in another, at the same instant becomes a stranger to him and separates from his body; so that the male recovers his individuality intact at the moment when he transcends it. The egg, on the contrary, begins to separate from the female body when, fully matured, it emerges from the follicle and falls into the oviduct; but if fertilised by a gamete from outside, it becomes attached again through implantation in the uterus. First violated, the female is then alienated – she becomes, in part, another than herself. She carries the foetus inside her abdomen until it reaches a stage of development that varies according to the species – the guinea-pig is born almost adult, the kangaroo still almost an embryo. Tenanted by another, who battens upon her substance throughout the period of pregnancy, the female is at once herself and other than herself; and after the birth she feeds the newborn upon the milk of her breasts. Thus it is not too clear when the new individual is to be regarded as autonomous: at the moment of fertilisation, of birth, or of weaning? It is noteworthy that the more clearly the female appears as a separate individual, the more imperiously the continuity of life asserts itself against her separateness. The fish and the bird, which expel the egg from the body before the embryo develops, are less enslaved to their offspring than is the female mammal. She regains some autonomy after the birth of her offspring – a certain distance is established between her and them; and it is following upon a separation that she devotes herself to them. She displays initiative and inventiveness in their behalf; she battles to defend them against other animals and may even become aggressive. But normally she does not seek to affirm her individuality; she is not hostile to males or to other females and shows little combative instinct. [Certain fowls wrangle over the best places in the poultry-yard and establish a hierarchy of dominance (the 'peck-order'); and sometimes among cattle there are cows that will fight for the leadership of the herd in the absence of males.] In spite of Darwin's theory of sexual selection, now much disputed, she accepts without discrimination whatever male happens to be at hand. It is not that the female lacks individual abilities – quite the contrary. At times when she is free from maternal servitude she can now and then equal the male; the mare is as fleet as the stallion, the hunting bitch has as keen a nose as the dog, she-monkeys in tests show as much intelligence as males. It is only that this individuality is not laid claim to; the female renounces it for the benefit of the species, which demands this abdication.

The lot of the male is quite different. As we have just seen, even in his transcendence towards the next generation he keeps himself apart and maintains his individuality within himself. This characteristic is constant, from the insect to the highest animals. Even in the fishes and whales, which live peaceably in mixed schools, the males separate from the rest at the time of rut, isolate themselves, and become aggressive towards other males. Immediate, direct in the female, sexuality is indirect, it is experienced through intermediate circumstances, in the male. There is a distance between desire and satisfaction which he actively surmounts; he pushes, seeks out, touches the female, caresses and quiets her before he penetrates her. The organs used in such activities are, as I have remarked, often better developed in the male than in the female. It is notable that the living impulse that brings about the vast production of sperms is expressed also in the male by the appearance of bright plumage, brilliant scales, horns, antlers, a mane, by his voice, his exuberance. We no longer believe that the 'wedding finery' put on by the male during rut, nor his seductive posturings, have selective significance; but they do manifest the power of life, bursting forth in him with useless and magnificent splendour. This vital superabundance, the activities directed towards mating, and the dominating affirmation of his power over the female in coitus itself – all this contributes to the assertion of the male individual as such at the moment of his living transcendence. In this respect Hegel is right in seeing the subjective element in the male, while the female remains wrapped up in the species. Subjectivity and separateness immediately signify conflict. Aggressiveness is one of the traits of the rutting male; and it is not explained by competition for mates, since the number of females is about equal to the number of males; it is rather the competition that is explained by this will to combat. It might be said that before procreating, the male claims as his own the act that perpetuates the species, and in doing battle with his peers confirms the truth of his individuality. The species takes residence in the female and absorbs most of her individual life; the male on the contrary integrates the specific vital forces into his individual life. No doubt he also submits to powers beyond his control: the sperms are formed within him and periodically he feels the rutting urge; but these processes involve the sum total of the organism in much less degree than does the oestrus cycle. The production of sperms is not exhausting, nor is the actual production of eggs; it is the development of the fertilised egg inside an adult animal that constitutes for the female an engrossing task. Coition is a rapid operation and one that robs the male of little vitality. He displays almost no paternal instinct. Very often he abandons the female after copulation. When he remains near her as head of a family group – monogamic family, harem, or herd – he nurtures and protects the community as a whole; only rarely does he take a direct interest in the young. In the species capable of high individual development, the urge of the male towards autonomy – which in lower animals is his ruin – is crowned with success. He is in general larger than the female, stronger, swifter, more adventurous; he leads a more independent life, his activities are more spontaneous; he is more masterful, more imperious. In mammalian societies it is always he who commands.

In nature nothing is ever perfectly dear. The two types, male and female, are not always sharply distinguished; while they sometimes exhibit a dimorphism – in coat colour or in arrangement of spotting or mottling – that seems absolutely distinctive, yet it may happen, on the contrary, that they are indistinguishable and that even their functions are hardly differentiated, as in many fishes. All in all, however, and especially at the top of the animal scale, the two sexes represent two diverse aspects of the life of the species. The difference between them is not, as has been claimed, that between activity and passivity; for the nucleus of the egg is active and moreover the development of the embryo is an active, living process, not a mechanical unfolding. It would be too simple to define the difference as that between change and permanence: for the sperm can create only because its vitality is maintained in the fertilised egg, and the egg can persist only through developmental change, without which it deteriorates and disappears.

It is true, however, that in these two processes, *maintaining* and *creating* (both of which are active), the synthesis of becoming is not accomplished in the same manner. To *maintain* is to deny the scattering of instants, it is to establish continuity in their flow; to *create* is to strike out from temporal unity in general an irreducible, separate present. And it is true also that in the female it is the continuity of life that seeks accomplishment in spite of separation; while separation into new and individualised forces is incited by male initiative. The male is thus permitted to express himself freely; the energy of the species is well integrated into his own living activity. On the contrary, the individuality of the female is opposed by the interest of the species; it is as if she were possessed by foreign forces – alienated. And this explains why the contrast between the sexes is not reduced when – as in higher forms – the individuality of the organisms concerned is more pronounced. On the contrary, the contrast is increased. The male finds more and more varied ways in which to employ the forces he is master of; the female feels her enslavement more and more keenly, the conflict between her own interests and the reproductive forces is heightened. Parturition in cows and mares is much more painful and dangerous than it is in mice and rabbits. Woman – the most individualised of females – seems to be the most fragile, most subject to this pain and danger: she who most dramatically fulfils the call of destiny and most profoundly differs from her male.

In man as in most animals the sexes are born in approximately equal numbers, the sex ratio for Western man being about 105.5 males to 100 females. Embryological development is analogous in the two sexes; however, in the female embryo the primitive germinal epithelium (from which ovary or testis develops) remains neutral longer and is therefore under the hormonal influence for a longer time, with the result that its development may be more often reversed. Thus it may be that the majority of pseudo-hermaphrodites are genotypically female subjects that have later become masculinised. One might suppose that the male organisation is defined as such at the beginning, whereas the female embryo is slower in taking on its femininity; but these early phenomena of foetal life are still too little known to permit of any certainty in interpretation.

Once established, the genital systems correspond in the two sexes, and the sex hormones of both belong to the same chemical group, that of the sterols; all are derived in the last analysis from cholesterol. They regulate the secondary sexual differences of the soma. Neither the chemical formulae of the hormones nor the anatomical peculiarities are sufficient to define the human female as such. It is her functional development that distinguishes her especially from the male.

The development of the male is comparatively simple. From birth to puberty his growth is almost regular; at the age of fifteen or sixteen spermatogenesis begins, and it continues into old age; with its appearance hormones are produced that establish the masculine bodily traits. From this point on, the male sex life is normally integrated with his individual existence: in desire and in coition his transcendence towards the species is at one with his subjectivity – he is his body.

Woman's story is much more complex. In embryonic life the supply of oocytes is already built up, the ovary containing about 40,000 immature eggs, each in a follicle, of which perhaps 400 will ultimately reach maturation. From birth, the species has taken possession of woman and tends to tighten its grasp. In coming into the world woman experiences a kind of first puberty, as the oocytes enlarge suddenly; then the ovary is reduced to about a fifth of its former size – one might say that the child is granted a respite. While her body develops, her genital system remains almost stationary; some of the follicles enlarge, but they fail to mature. The growth of the little girl is similar to that of the boy; at the same age she is sometimes even taller and heavier than he is. But at puberty the species reasserts its claim. Under the influence of the ovarian secretions the number of developing follicles increases, the ovary receives more blood and grows larger, one of the follicles matures, ovulation occurs, and the menstrual cycle is initiated; the genital system assumes its definitive size and form, the body takes on feminine contours, and the endocrine balance is established.

It is to be noted that this whole occurrence has the aspect of a *crisis*. Not without resistance does the body of woman permit the species to take over; and this struggle is weakening and dangerous. Before puberty almost as many boys die as girls; from age fourteen to eighteen, 128 girls die to 100 boys, and from eighteen to twenty-two, 105 girls to 100 boys. At this period frequently appear such diseases as chlorosis tuberculosis, scoliosis (curvature of the spine), and osteomyelitis (inflammation of the bone marrow). In some cases puberty is abnormally precocious, appearing as early as age four or five. In others, on the contrary puberty fails to become established, the subject remaining infantile and suffering from disorders of menstruation (amenorrhea or dysmenorrhea). Certain women show signs of virilism, taking on masculine traits as a result of excessive adrenal secretion.

Such abnormalities in no way represent victories of the individual over the species; there is no way of escape, for as it enslaves the individual life, the species simultaneously supports and nourishes it. This duality is expressed at the level of the ovarian functions, since the vitality of woman has its roots in the ovaries as that of man in the testicles. In both sexes a castrated individual is not merely sterile; he or she suffers regression, degenerates. Not properly constituted, the whole organism is impoverished and thrown out of balance; it can expand and flourish only as its genital system expands and flourishes. And furthermore many reproductive phenomena are unconcerned with the individual life of the subject and may even be sources of danger. The mammary glands, developing at puberty, play no role in woman's individual economy: they can be excised at any time of life. Many of the ovarian secretions function for the benefit of the egg, promoting its maturation and adapting the uterus to its requirements; in respect to the organism as a whole they make for disequilibration rather than for regulation – the woman is adapted to the needs of the egg rather than to her own requirements.

From puberty to menopause woman is the theatre of a play that unfolds within her and in which she is not personally concerned. Anglo-Saxons call menstruation 'the curse'; in truth the menstrual cycle is a burden, and a useless one from the point of view of the individual. In Aristotle's time it was believed that each month blood flowed away that was intended, if fertilisation had occurred, to build up the blood and flesh of the infant, and the truth of that old notion lies in the fact that over and over again woman does sketch in outline the groundwork of gestation. In lower mammals this oestrus cycle is confined to a particular season, and it is not accompanied by a flow of blood; only in the primates (monkeys, apes, and the human species) is it marked each month by blood and more or less pain. ['Analysis of these phenomena in recent years has shown that they are similar in woman and the higher monkeys and apes, especially in the genus Rhesus. It *is evidently easier* to experiment with *these animals*,' writes Louis Callien (*La Sexualité*).] During about fourteen days one of the Graafian follicles that enclose the eggs enlarges and matures, secreting the hormone folliculin (estrin). Ovulation occurs on about the fourteenth day: the follicle protrudes through the surface of the ovary and breaks open (sometimes with slight bleeding), the egg passes into the oviduct, and the wound develops into the corpus luteum. The latter secretes the hormone progesterone, which acts on the uterus during the second phase of the cycle. The lining of the uterus becomes thickened and glandular and full of blood vessels, forming in the womb a cradle to receive the fertilised egg. These cellular proliferations being irreversible, the edifice is not resorbed if fertilisation has not occurred. In the lower mammals the debris may escape gradually or may be carried away by the lymphatic vessels; but in woman and the other primates, the thickened lining membrane (endometrium) breaks down suddenly, the blood vessels and blood spaces are opened, and the bloody mass trickles out as the menstrual flow. Then, while the corpus luteum regresses, the membrane that lines the uterus is reconstituted and a new follicular phase of the cycle begins.

This complex process, still mysterious in many of its details, involves the whole female organism, since there are hormonal reactions between the ovaries and other endocrine organs, such as the pituitary, the thyroid, and the adrenals, which affect the central nervous system, the sympathetic nervous system, and in consequence all the viscera. Almost all women – more than 85 per cent – show more or less distressing symptoms during the menstrual period. Blood pressure rises before the beginning of the flow and falls afterwards; the pulse rate and often the temperature are increased, so that fever is frequent; pains in the abdomen are felt; often a tendency to constipation followed by diarrhoea is observed; frequently there are also swelling of the liver, retention of urea, and albuminuria; many subjects have sore throat and difficulties with hearing and sight; perspiration is increased and accompanied at the beginning of the menses by an odour *sui generis*, which may be very strong and may persist throughout the period. The rate of basal metabolism is raised. The red blood count drops. The blood carries substances usually put on reserve in the tissues, especially calcium salts; the presence of these substances reacts on the ovaries, on the thyroid – which enlarges – and on the pituitary (regulator of the changes in the uterine lining described above) more active. This glandular instability brings on a pronounced nervous instability. The central nervous system is affected, with frequent headache, and the sympathetic system is overactive; unconscious control through the central system is reduced, freeing convulsive reflexes and complexes and leading to a marked capriciousness of disposition. The woman is more emotional, more nervous, more irritable than usual, and may manifest serious psychic disturbance. It is during her periods that she feels her body most painfully as an obscure, alien thing; it is, indeed, the prey of a stubborn and foreign life that each month constructs and then tears down a cradle within it; each month all things are made ready for a child and then aborted in the crimson flow. Woman, like man, is her body; ['So I am body, in so far, at least, as my experience goes, and conversely a life-model, or like a preliminary sketch, for my total being.' Merleau-Ponty, *Phénoménologie de la perception*.] but her body is something other than herself.

Woman experiences a more profound alienation when fertilisation has occurred and the dividing egg passes down into the uterus and proceeds to develop there. True enough, pregnancy is a normal process, which, if it takes place under normal conditions of health and nutrition, is not harmful to the mother; certain interactions between her and the foetus become established which are even beneficial to her. In spite of an optimistic view having all too obvious social utility, however, gestation is a fatiguing task of no individual benefit to the woman [I am taking here an exclusively physiological point of view. It is evident that maternity can be very advantageous psychologically for a woman, just as it can also be a disaster.] but on the contrary demanding heavy sacrifices. It is often associated in the first months with loss of appetite and vomiting, which are not observed in any female domesticated animal and which signalise the revolt of the organism against the invading species. There is a loss of phosphorus, calcium, and iron – the last difficult to make good later; metabolic overactivity excites the endocrine system; the sympathetic nervous system is in a state of increased excitement; and the blood shows a lowered specific gravity, it is lacking in iron, and in general it is similar 'to that of persons fasting, of victims of famine, of those who have been bled frequently, of convalescents'. All that a healthy and well-nourished woman can hope for is to recoup these losses without too much difficulty after childbirth; but frequently serious accidents or at least dangerous disorders mark the course of pregnancy; and if the woman is not strong, if hygienic precautions are not taken, repeated child-bearing will make her prematurely old and misshapen, as often among the rural poor. Childbirth itself is painful and dangerous. In this crisis it is most clearly evident that the body does not always work to the advantage of both species and individual at once; the infant may die, and, again, in being born it may kill its mother or leave her with a chronic ailment. Nursing is also a tiring service. A number of factors – especially the hormone prolactin bring about the secretion of milk in the mammary glands; some soreness and often fever may accompany the process and in any case the nursing mother feeds the newborn from the resources of her own vitality. The conflict between species and individual, which sometimes assumes dramatic force at childbirth, endows the feminine body with a disturbing frailty. It has been well said that women 'have infirmity in the abdomen'; and it is true that they have within them a hostile element – it is the species gnawing at their vitals. Their maladies are often caused not by some infection from without but by some internal maladjustment; for example, a false inflammation of the endometrium is set up through the reaction of the uterine lining to an abnormal excitation of the ovaries; if the corpus luteum persists instead of declining menstruation, it causes inflammation of the oviducts and uterine lining, and so on.

In the end woman escapes the iron grasp of the species by way of still another serious crisis; the phenomena of the menopause, the inverse of puberty, appear between the ages of forty-five and fifty. Ovarian activity diminishes and disappears, with resulting impoverishment of the individual's vital forces. It may be supposed that the metabolic glands, the thyroid and pituitary, are compelled to make up in some fashion for the functioning of the ovaries; and thus, along with the depression natural to the change of life, are to be noted signs excitation, such as high blood pressure, hot flushes, nervousness, and sometimes increased sexuality. Some women develop fat deposits at this time; others become masculinised. In many, a new endocrine balance becomes established. Woman is now delivered from the servitude imposed by her female nature, but she is not to be likened to a eunuch, for her vitality is unimpaired. And what is more, she is no longer the prey of overwhelming forces; she is herself, she and her body are one. It is sometimes said that women of a certain age constitute 'a third sex'; and, in truth, while they are not males, they are no longer females. Often, indeed, this release from female physiology is expressed in a health, a balance, a vigour that they lacked before.

In addition to the primary sexual characteristics, woman has various secondary sexual peculiarities that are more or less directly produced in consequence of the first, through hormonal action. On the average she is shorter than the male and lighter, her skeleton is more delicate, and the pelvis is larger in adaptation to the functions of pregnancy and childbirth; her connective tissues accumulate fat and her contours are thus more rounded than those of the male. Appearance in general – structure, skin, hair – is distinctly different in the two sexes. Muscular strength is much less in woman, about two thirds that of man; she has less respiratory capacity, the lungs and trachea being smaller. The larynx is relatively smaller, and in consequence the female voice is higher. The specific gravity of the blood is lower in woman and there is less haemoglobin; women are therefore less robust and more disposed to anaemia than are males. Their pulse is more rapid, the vascular system less stable, with ready blushing. Instability is strikingly characteristic of woman's organisation in general; among other things, man shows greater stability in the metabolism of calcium, woman fixing much less of this material and losing a good deal during menstruation and pregnancy. It would seem that in regard to calcium the ovaries exert a catabolic action, with resulting instability that brings on difficulties in the ovaries and in the thyroid, which is more developed in woman than in man. Irregularities in the endocrine secretions react on the sympathetic nervous system, and nervous and muscular control is uncertain. This lack in stability and control underlies woman's emotionalism, which is bound up with circulatory fluctuations palpitation of the heart, blushing, and so forth – and on this account women are subject to such displays of agitation as tears, hysterical laughter, and nervous crises.

It is obvious once more that many of these traits originate in woman's subordination to the species, and here we find the most striking conclusion of this survey: namely, that woman is of all mammalian females at once the one who is most profoundly alienated (her individuality the prey of outside forces), and the one who most violently resists this alienation; in no other is enslavement of the organism to reproduction more imperious or more unwillingly accepted. Crises of puberty and the menopause, monthly 'curse', long and often difficult pregnancy, painful and sometimes dangerous childbirth, illnesses, unexpected symptoms and complications – these are characteristic of the human female. It would seem that her lot is heavier than that of other females in just about the same degree that she goes beyond other females in the assertion of her individuality. In comparison with her the male seems infinitely favoured: his sexual life is not in opposition to his existence as a person, and biologically it runs an even course, without crises and generally without mishap. On the average, women live as long as men, or longer; but they are much more often ailing, and there are many times when they are not in command of themselves.

These biological considerations are extremely important. In the history of woman they play a part of the first rank and constitute an essential element in her situation. Throughout our further discussion we shall always bear them in mind. For, the body being the instrument of our grasp upon the world, the world is bound to seem a very different thing when apprehended in one manner or another. This accounts for our lengthy study of the biological facts; they are one of the kys to the understanding of woman. But I deny that they establish for her a fixed and inevitable destiny. They are insufficient for setting up a hierarchy of the sexes; they fail to explain why woman is the Other; they do not condemn her to remain in this subordinate role for ever.

It has been frequently maintained that in physiology alone must be sought the answers to these questions: Are the chances for individual success the same in the two sexes? Which plays the more important role in the species? But it must be noted that the first of these problems is quite different in the case of woman, as compared with other females; for animal species are fixed and it is possible to define them in static terms – by merely collecting observations it can be decided whether the mare is as fast as the stallion, or whether male chimpanzees excel their mates in intelligence tests – whereas the human species is for ever in a state of change, for ever becoming.

Certain materialist savants have approached the problem in a purely static fashion; influenced by the theory of psychophysiological parallelism, they sought to work out mathematical comparisons between the male and female organism – and they imagined that these measurements registered directly the functional capacities of the two sexes. For example, these students have engaged in elaborately trifling discussions regarding the absolute and relative weight of the brain in man and woman – with inconclusive results, after all corrections have been made. But what destroys much of the interest of these careful researches is the fact that it has not been possible to establish any relation whatever between the weight of the brain and the level of intelligence. And one would similarly be at a loss to present a psychic interpretation of the chemical formulae designating the male and female hormones.

As for the present study, I categorically reject the notion of psychophysiological parallelism, for it is a doctrine whose foundations have long since been thoroughly undermined. If I mention it at all, it is because it still haunts many minds in spite of its philosophical and scientific bankruptcy. I reject also any comparative system that assumes the existence of a natural hierarchy or scale of values – for example, an evolutionary hierarchy. It is vain to ask if the female body is or is not more infantile than that of the male, if it is more or less similar to that of the apes, and so on. All these dissertations which mingle a vague naturalism with a still more vague ethics or aesthetics are pure verbiage. It is only in a human perspective that we can compare the female and the male of the human species. But man is defined as a being who is not fixed, who makes himself what he is. As Merleau-Ponty very justly puts it, man is not a natural species: he is a historical idea. Woman is not a completed reality, but rather a becoming, and it is in her becoming that she should be compared with man; that is to say, her possibilities should be defined. What gives rise to much of the debate is the tendency to reduce her to what she has been, to what she is today, in raising the question of her capabilities; for the fact is that capabilities are clearly manifested only when they have been realised – but the fact is also that when we have to do with a being whose nature is transcendent action, we can never close the books.

Nevertheless it will be said that if the body is not a thing, it is a situation, as viewed in the perspective I am adopting – that of Heidegger, Sartre, and Merleau-Ponty: it is the instrument of our grasp upon the world, a limiting factor for our projects. Woman is weaker than man, she has less muscular strength, fewer red blood corpuscles, less lung capacity, she runs more slowly, can lift less heavy weights, can compete with man in hardly any sport; she cannot stand up to him in a fight. To all this weakness must be added the instability, the lack of control, and the fragility already discussed: these are facts. Her grasp on the world is thus more restricted; she has less firmness and less steadiness available for projects that in general she is less capable of carrying out. In other words, her individual life is less rich than man's.

Certainly these facts cannot be denied – but in themselves they have no significance. Once we adopt the human perspective, interpreting the body on a basis of existence, biology becomes an abstract science; whenever the physiological fact (for instance, muscular inferiority) takes on meaning, this meaning is at once seen as dependent on a whole context; the 'weakness' is revealed as such only in the light of the ends man proposes, the instruments he has available, and the laws he establishes. If he does not wish to seize the world, then the idea of a *grasp* on things has no sense; when in this seizure the full employment of bodily power is not required, above the available minimum, then differences in strength are annulled; wherever violence is contrary to custom, muscular force cannot be a basis for domination. In brief, the concept of *weakness* can be defined only with reference to existentialist, economic, and moral considerations. It has been said that the human species is anti-natural, a statement that is hardly exact, since man cannot deny facts; but he establishes their truth by the way in which he deals with them; nature has reality for him only to the extent that it is involved in his activity – his own nature not excepted. As with her grasp on the world, it is again impossible to measure in the abstract the burden imposed on woman by her reproductive function. The bearing of maternity upon the individual life, regulated naturally in animals by the oestrus cycle and the seasons, is not definitely prescribed in woman – society alone is the arbiter. The bondage of woman to the species is more or less rigorous according to the number of births demanded by society and the degree of hygienic care provided for pregnancy and childbirth. Thus, while it is true that in the higher animals the individual existence is asserted more imperiously by the male than by the female, in the human species individual 'possibilities' depend upon the economic and social situation.

But in any case it does not always happen that the male's individual privileges give him a position of superiority within the species, for in maternity the female acquires a kind of autonomy of her own. Sometimes, as in the baboons studied by Zuckermann, [*The Social Life of Monkeys and Apes* (1932).] the male does dominate; but in many species the two members of the pair lead a separate life, and in the lion the two sexes share equally in the duties the den. Here again the human situation cannot be reduced to any other; it is not as single individuals that human beings are to be defined in the first place; men and women have never stood opposed to each other in single combat; the couple is an original *Mitsein*, a basic combination; and as such it always appears as a permanent or temporary element in a large collectivity.

Within such a society, which is more necessary to the species, male or female? At the level of the gametes, at the level of the biological functions of coition and pregnancy, the male principle creates to maintain, the female principle maintains to create, as we have seen; but what are the various aspects of this division of labour in different forms of social life? In sessile species, attached to other organisms or to substrata, in those furnished by nature with abundant sustenance obtainable without effort, the role of the male is limited to fecundation; where it is necessary to seek, to hunt, to fight in order to provide the food needed by the young, the male in many cases co-operates in their support. This co-operation becomes absolutely indispensable in a species where the offspring remain unable to take care of themselves for a long time after weaning; here the male's assistance becomes extremely important, for the lives he has begotten cannot be maintained without him. A single male can fecundate a number of females each year; but it requires a male for every female to assure the survival of the offspring after they are born, to defend them against enemies, to wrest from nature the wherewithal to satisfy their needs. In human history the equilibrium between the forces of production and of reproduction is brought about by different means under different economic conditions, and these conditions govern the relations of male and female to offspring and in consequence to each other. But here we are leaving the realm of biology; by its light alone we could never decide the primacy of one sex or the other in regard to the perpetuation of the species.

But in truth a society is not a species, for it is in a society that the species attains the status of existence – transcending itself towards the world and towards the future. Its ways and customs cannot be deduced from biology, for the individuals that compose the society are never abandoned to the dictates of their nature; they are subject rather to that second nature which is custom and in which are reflected the desires and the fears that express their essential nature. It is not merely as a body, but rather as a body subject to taboos, to laws, that the subject is conscious of himself and attains fulfilment – it is with reference to certain values that he evaluates himself. And, once again, it is not upon physiology that values can be based; rather, the facts of biology take on the values that the existent bestows upon them. If the respect or the fear inspired by woman prevents the use of violence towards her, then the muscular superiority of the male is no source of power. If custom decrees – as in certain Indian tribes – that the young girls are to choose their husbands, or if the father dictates the marriage choice, then the sexual aggressiveness of the male gives him no power of initiative, no advantage. The close bond between mother and child will be for her a source of dignity or indignity according to the value placed upon the child – which is highly variable this very bond, as we have seen, will be recognised or not according to the presumptions of the society concerned.

Thus we must view the facts of biology in the light of an ontological, economic, social, and psychological context. The enslavement of the female to the species and the limitations of her various powers are extremely important facts; the body of woman is one of the essential elements in her situation in the world. But that body is not enough to define her as woman; there is no true living reality except as manifested by the conscious individual through activities and in the bosom of a society. Biology is not enough to give an answer to the question that is before us: why is woman the Other? Our task is to discover how the nature of woman has been affected throughout the course of history; we are concerned to find out what humanity has made of the human female.

The Second Sex
by Simone de Beauvoir (1949)

Book One: Facts and Myths, Part I: Destiny

Chapter 2: The Psychoanalytic Point of View

THE tremendous advance accomplished by psychoanalysis over psychophysiology lies in the view that no factor becomes involved in the psychic life without having taken on human significance; it is not the body-object described by biologists that actually exists, but the body as lived by the subject. Woman is a female to the extent that she feels herself as such. There are biologically essential features that are not a part of her real, experienced situation: thus the structure of the egg is not reflected in it, but on the contrary an organ of no great biological importance, like the clitoris, plays in it a part of the first rank. It is not nature that defines woman; it is she who defines herself by dealing with nature on her own account in her emotional life.

An entire system has been built up in this perspective, which I do not intend to criticise as a whole, merely examining its contribution to the study of woman. It is not an easy matter to discuss psychoanalysis *per se*. Like all religions – Christianity and Marxism, for example – it displays an embarrassing flexibility on a basis of rigid concepts. Words are sometimes used in their most literal sense, the term *phallus*, for example, designating quite exactly that fleshy projection which marks the male; again, they are indefinitely expanded and take on symbolic meaning, the phallus now expressing the virile character and situation *in toto*. If you attack the letter of his doctrine, the psychoanalyst protests that you misunderstand its spirit; if you applaud its spirit, he at once wishes to confine you to the letter. The doctrine is of no importance, says one, psychoanalysis is a method; but the success of the method strengthens the doctrinaire in his faith. After all, where is one to find the true lineaments of psychoanalysis if not among the psychoanalysts? But there are heretics among these, just as there are among Christians and Marxists; and more than one psychoanalyst has declared that 'the worst enemies of psychoanalysis are the psychoanalysts'. In spite of a scholastic precision that often becomes pedantic, many obscurities remain to be dissipated. As Sartre and Merleau-Ponty have observed, the proposition 'Sexuality is coextensive with existence' can be understood in two very different ways; it can mean that every experience of the existent has a sexual significance, or that every sexual phenomenon has an existential import. It is possible to reconcile these statements, but too often one merely slips from one to the other. Furthermore, as soon as the 'sexual' is distinguished from the 'genital', the idea of sexuality becomes none too clear. According to Dalbiez, 'the sexual with Freud is the intrinsic aptitude for releasing the genital'. But nothing is more obscure than the idea of 'aptitude' – that is, of possibility – for only realisation gives indubitable proof of what is possible. Not being a philosopher, Freud has refused to justify his system philosophically; and his disciples maintain that on this account he is exempt from all metaphysical attack. There are metaphysical assumptions behind all his dicta, however, and to use his language is to adopt a philosophy. It is just such confusions that call for criticism, while making criticism difficult.

Freud never showed much concern with the destiny of woman; it is clear that he simply adapted his account from that of the destiny of man, with slight modifications. Earlier the sexologist Marañon had stated that 'As specific energy, we may say that the libido is a force of virile character. We will say as much of the orgasm'. According to him, women who attain orgasm are 'viriloid' women; the sexual impulse is 'in one direction' and woman is only half way along the road. Freud never goes to such an extreme; he admits that woman's sexuality is evolved as fully as man's; but he hardly studies it in particular. He writes: 'The libido is constantly and regularly male in essence, whether it appears in man or in woman.' He declines to regard the feminine libido as having its own original nature, and therefore it will necessarily seem to him like a complex deviation from the human libido in general. This develops at first, he thinks, identically in the two sexes – each infant passes first through an oral phase that fixates it upon the maternal breast, and then through an anal phase; finally it reaches the genital phase, at which point the sexes become differentiated.

Freud further brought to light a fact the importance of which had not been fully appreciated: namely, that masculine erotism is definitely located in the penis, whereas in woman there are two distinct erotic systems: one the clitoral, which develops in childhood, the other vaginal, which develops only after puberty. When the boy reaches the genital phase, his evolution is completed, though he must pass from the auto-erotic inclination, in which pleasure is subjective, to the hetero-erotic inclination, in which pleasure is bound up with an object, normally a woman. This transition is made at the time of puberty through a narcissistic phase. But the penis will remain, as in childhood, the specific organ of erotism. Woman's libido, also passing through a narcissistic phase, will become objective, normally towards man; but the process will be much more complex, because woman must pass from clitoral pleasure to vaginal. There is only one genital stage for man, but there are two for woman; she runs a much greater risk of not reaching the end of her sexual evolution, of remaining at the infantile stage and thus of developing neuroses.

While still in the auto-erotic stage, the child becomes more or less strongly attached to an object. The boy becomes fixed on his mother and desires to identify himself with his father; this presumption terrifies him and he dreads mutilation at the hands of his father in punishment for it. Thus the castration complex springs from the Oedipus complex. Then aggressiveness towards the father develops, but at the same time the child interiorises the father's authority; thus the superego is built up in the child and censures his incestuous tendencies. These are repressed, the complex is liquidated, and the son is freed from his fear of his father, whom he has now installed in his own psyche under the guise of moral precepts. The super-ego is more powerful in proportion as the Oedipus complex has been more marked and more rigorously resisted.

Freud at first described the little girl's history in a completely corresponding fashion, later calling the feminine form of the process the Electra complex; but it is clear that he defined it less in itself than upon the basis of his masculine pattern. He recognised a very important difference between the two, however: the little girl at first has a mother fixation, but the boy is at no time sexually attracted to the father. This fixation of the girl represents a survival of the oral phase. Then the child identifies herself with the father; but towards the age of five she discovers the anatomical difference between the sexes, and she reacts to the absence of the penis by acquiring a castration complex – she imagines that she has been mutilated and is pained at the thought. Having then to renounce her virile pretensions, she identifies herself with her mother and seeks to seduce the father. The castration complex and the Electra complex thus reinforce each other. Her feeling of frustration is the keener since, loving her father, she wishes in vain to be like him; and, inversely, her regret strengthens her love, for she is able to compensate for her inferiority through the affection she inspires in her father. The little girl entertains a feeling of rivalry and hostility towards her mother. Then the super-ego is built up also in her, and the incestuous tendencies are repressed; but her super-ego is not so strong, for the Electra complex is less sharply defined than the Oedipus because the first fixation was upon the mother, and since the father is himself the object of the love that he condemns, his prohibitions are weaker than in the case of his son-rival. It can be seen that like her genital development the whole sexual drama is more complex for the girl than for her brothers. In consequence she may be led to react to the castration complex by denying her femininity, by continuing obstinately to covet a penis and to identify herself with her father. This attitude will cause her to remain in the clitoral phase, to become frigid or to turn towards homosexuality.

The two essential objections that may be raised against this view derive from the fact that Freud based it upon a masculine model. He assumes that woman feels that she is a mutilated man. But the idea of mutilation implies comparison and evaluation. Many psychoanalysts today admit that the young girl may regret not having a penis without believing, however, that it has been removed from her body, and even this regret is not general. It could not arise from a simple anatomical comparison; many little girls, in fact, are late in discovering the masculine construction, and if they do, it is only by sight. The little boy obtains from his penis a living experience that makes it an object of pride to him, but this pride does not necessarily imply a corresponding humiliation for his sisters, since they know the masculine organ in its outward aspect only – this outgrowth, this weak little rod of flesh can in itself only inspire them only with indifference, or even disgust. The little girl's covetousness, when it exists, results from a previous evaluation of virility. Freud takes this for granted, when it should be accounted for. On the other hand, the concept of the Electra complex is very vague, because it is not supported by a basic description of the feminine libido. Even in boys the occurrence of a definitely genital Oedipus complex is by no means general; but, apart from very few exceptions, it cannot be admitted that the father is a source of genital excitation for his young daughter. One of the great problems of feminine eroticism is that clitoral pleasure is localised; and it is only towards puberty that a number of erogenous zones develop in various parts of the body, along with the growth of vaginal sensation. To say, then, that in a child of ten the kisses and caresses of her father have an 'intrinsic aptitude' for arousing clitoral pleasure is to assert something that in most cases is nonsense. If it is admitted that the Electra complex has only a very diffuse emotional character, then the whole question of emotion is raised, and Freudianism does not help us in defining emotion as distinguished from sexuality. What deifies the father is by no means the feminine libido (nor is the mother deified by the desire she arouses in the son); on the contrary, the fact that the feminine desire (in the daughter) is directed towards a sovereign being gives it a special character. It does not determine the nature of its object; rather it is affected by the latter. The sovereignty of the father is a fact of social origin, which Freud fails to account for; in fact, he states that it is impossible to say what authority decided, at a certain moment in history, that the father should take precedence over the mother – a decision that, according to Freud, was progressive, but due to causes unknown. 'It could not have been patriarchal authority, since it is just this authority which progress conferred upon the father', as he puts it in his last work.

Adler took issue with Freud because he saw the deficiency of a system that undertook to explain human life upon the basis of sexuality alone; he holds that sexuality should be integrated with the total personality. With Freud all human behaviour seems to be the outcome of desire – that is, of the search for pleasure – but for Adler man appears to be aiming at certain goals; for the sexual urge he substitutes motives, purposes, projects. He gives so large a place to the intelligence that often the sexual has in his eyes only a symbolic value. According to his system, the human drama can be reduced to three elemental factors: in every individual there is a will to power, which, however, is accompanied by an inferiority complex; the resulting conflict leads the individual to employ a thousand ruses in a flight from reality – a reality with which he fears he may not be able to cope; the subject thus withdraws to some degree from the society of which he is apprehensive and hence becomes afflicted with the neuroses that involve disturbance of the social attitude. In woman the inferiority complex takes the form of a shamed rejection of her femininity. It is not the lack of the penis that causes this complex, but rather woman's total situation; if the little girl feels penis envy it is only as the symbol of privileges enjoyed by boys. The place the father holds in the family, the universal predominance of males, her own education – everything confirms her in her belief in masculine superiority. Later on, when she takes part in sexual relations, she finds a new humiliation in the coital posture that places woman underneath the man. She reacts through the 'masculine protest': either she endeavours to masculinise herself, or she makes use of her feminine weapons to wage war upon the male. Through maternity she may be able to find an equivalent of the penis in her child. But this supposes that she begins by wholly accepting her role as woman and that she assumes her inferiority. She is divided against herself much more profoundly than is the male.

I shall not enlarge here upon the theoretical differences that separate Adler and Freud nor upon the possibilities of a reconciliation; but this may be said: neither the explanation based upon the sexual urge nor that based upon motive is sufficient, for every urge poses a motive, but the motive is apprehended only through the urge – a synthesis of Adlerianism and Freudianism would therefore seem possible of realisation. In fact, Adler retains the idea of psychic causation as an integral part of his system when he introduces the concepts of goal and of fiality, and he is somewhat in accord with Freud in regard to the relation between drives and mechanism: the physicist always recognises determinism when he is concerned with conflict or a force of attraction. The axiomatic proposition held in common by all psychoanalysts is this: the human story is to be explained by the interplay of determinate elements. And all the psychoanalysts allot the same destiny to woman. Her drama is epitomised in the conflict between her 'viriloid' and her 'feminine' tendencies, the first expressed through the clitoral system, the second in vaginal erotism. As a child she identifies herself with her father; then she becomes possessed with a feeling of inferiority with reference to the male and is faced with a dilemma: either to assert her independence and become virilised – which, with the underlying complex of inferiority, induces a state of tension that threatens neurosis – or to find happy fulfilment in amorous submission, a solution that is facilitated by her love for the sovereign father. He it is whom she really seeks in lover or husband, and thus her sexual love is mingled with the desire to be dominated. She will find her recompense in maternity, since that will afford her a new kind of independence. This drama would seem to be endowed with an energy, dynamism, of its own; it steadily pursues its course through any and all distorting incidents, and every woman is passively swept along in it.

The psychoanalysts have had no trouble in finding empirical confirmation for their theories. As we know, it was possible for a long time to explain the position of the planets on the Ptolemaic system by adding to it sufficiently subtle complications; and by superposing an inverse Oedipus complex upon the Oedipus complex, by disclosing desire in all anxiety, success has been achieved in integrating with the Freudian system the very facts that appear to contradict its validity. It is possible to make out a form only against a background, and the way in which the form is apprehended brings out the background behind it in positive detail; thus, if one is determined to describe a special case in a Freudian perspective, one will encounter the Freudian schema behind it. But when a doctrine demands the indefinite and arbitrary multiplication of secondary explanations, when observation brings to light as many exceptions as instances conformable to rule, it is better to give up the old rigid framework. Indeed, every psychoanalyst today is busily engaged after his fashion in making the Freudian concepts less rigid and in attempting compromises. For example, a contemporary psychoanalyst [Baudouin] writes as follows:

'Wherever there is a complex, there are by definition a number of components ... The complex consists in the association of these disparate elements and not in the representation of one among them by the others.' But the concept of a simple association of elements is unacceptable, for the psychic life is not a mosaic, it is a single whole in every one of its aspects and we must respect that unity. This is possible only by our recovering through the disparate facts the original purposiveness of existence. If we do not go back to this source, man appears to be the battleground of compulsions and prohibitions that alike are devoid of meaning and incidental.

All psychoanalysts systematically reject the idea of choice and the correlated concept of value, and therein lies the intrinsic weakness of the system. Having dissociated compulsions and prohibitions from the free choice of the existent, Freud fails to give us an explanation of their origin – he takes them for granted. He endeavoured to replace the idea of value with that of authority; but he admits in *Moses and Monotheism* that he has no way of accounting for this authority. Incest, for example, is forbidden because the father has forbidden it – but why did he forbid it? It is a mystery. The super-ego interiorises, introjects commands and prohibitions emanating from an arbitrary tyranny, and the instinctive drives are there, we know not why: these two realities are unrelated because morality is envisaged as foreign to sexuality. The human unity appears to be disrupted, there is no thoroughfare from the individual to society; to reunite them Freud was forced to invent strange fictions, as in *Totem and Taboo*. Adler saw clearly that the castration complex could be explained only in social context; he grappled with the problem of valuation, but he did not reach the source in the individual of the values recognised by society, and he did not grasp that values are involved in sexuality itself, which led him to misjudge its importance.

Sexuality most certainly plays a considerable role in human life; it can be said to pervade life throughout. We have already learned from physiology that the living activity of the testes and the ovaries is integrated with that of the body in general. The existent is a sexual, a sexuate body, and in his relations with other existents who are also sexuate bodies, sexuality is in consequence always involved. But if body and sexuality are concrete expressions of existence, it is with reference to this that their significance can be discovered. Lacking this perspective, psychoanalysis takes for granted unexplained facts. For instance, we are told that the little girl is ashamed of urinating in a squatting position with her bottom uncovered – but whence comes this shame? And likewise, before asking whether the male is proud of having a penis or whether his pride is expressed in his penis, it is necessary to know what pride is and how the aspirations of the subject can be incarnated in an object. There is no need of taking sexuality as an irreducible datum, for there is in the existent a more original 'quest for being', of which sexuality is only one of the aspects. Sartre demonstrates this truth in *L'Être et le néant*, as does Bachelard in his works on Earth, Air, and Water. The psychoanalysts hold that the primary truth regarding man is his relation with his own body and with the bodies of his fellows in the group; but man has a primordial interest in the substance of the natural world which surrounds him and which he tries to discover in work, in play, and in all the experiences of the 'dynamic imagination'. Man aspires to be at one concretely with the whole world, apprehended in all possible ways. To work the earth, to dig a hole, are activities as original as the embrace, as coition, and they deceive themselves who see here no more than sexual symbols. The hole, the ooze, the gash, hardness, integrity are primary realities; and the interest they have for man is not dictated by the libido, but rather the libido will be coloured by the manner in which he becomes aware of them. It is not because it symbolises feminine virginity that integrity fascinates man; but it is his admiration for integrity that renders virginity precious. Work, war, play, art signify ways of being concerned with the world which cannot be reduced to any others; they disclose qualities that interfere with those which sexuality reveals. It is at once in their light and in the light of these erotic experiences that the individual exercises his power of choice. But only an ontological point of view, a comprehension of being in general, permits us to restore the unity of this choice.

It is this concept of choice, indeed, that psychoanalysis most vehemently rejects in the name of determinism and the 'collective unconscious'; and it is this unconscious that is supposed to supply man with prefabricated imagery and a universal symbolism. Thus it would explain the observed analogies of dreams, of purposeless actions, of visions of delirium, of allegories, and of human destinies. To speak of liberty would be to deny oneself the possibility of explaining these disturbing conformities. But the idea of liberty is not incompatible with the existence of certain constants. If the psychoanalytic method is frequently rewarding in spite of the errors in its theory, that is because there are in every individual case certain factors of undeniable generality: situations and behaviour patterns constantly recur, and the moment of decision flashes from a cloud of generality and repetition. 'Anatomy is destiny', said Freud; and this phrase is echoed by that of Merleau-Ponty: 'The body is generality.' Existence is all one, bridging the gaps between individual existents; it makes itself manifest in analogous organisms, and therefore constant factors will be found in the bonds between the ontological and the sexual. At a given epoch of history the techniques, the economic and social structure of a society, will reveal to all its members an identical world, and there a constant relation of sexuality to social patterns will exist; analogous individuals, placed in analogous conditions, will see analogous points of significance in the given circumstances. This analogy does not establish a rigorous universality, but it accounts for the fact that general types may be recognised in individual case histories.

The symbol does not seem to me to be an allegory elaborated by a mysterious unconscious; it is rather the perception of a certain significance through the analogue of the significant object. Symbolic significance is manifested in the same way to numerous individuals, because of the identical existential situation connecting all the individual existents, and the identical set of artificial conditions that all must confront. Symbolism did not come down from heaven nor rise up from subterranean depths – it has been elaborated, like language, by that human reality which is at once *Mitsein* and separation; and this explains why individual invention also has its place, as in practice psychoanalysis has to admit, regardless of doctrine. Our perspective allows us, for example, to understand the value widely accorded to the penis. It is impossible to account for it without taking our departure from an existential fact: the tendency of the subject towards *alienation*. The anxiety that his liberty induces in the subject leads him to search for himself in things, which is a kind of flight from himself. This tendency is so fundamental that immediately after weaning, when he is separated from the Whole, the infant is compelled to lay hold upon his alienated existence in mirrors and in the gaze of his parents. Primitive people are alienated in mana, in the totem; civilised people in their individual souls, in their egos, their names, their property, their work. Here is to be found the primary temptation to inauthenticity, to failure to be genuinely oneself. The penis is singularly adapted for playing this role of 'double' for the little boy – it is for him at once a foreign object and himself; it is a plaything, a doll, and yet his own flesh; relatives and nurse-girls behave towards it as if it were a little person. It is easy to see, then, how it becomes for the child 'an *alter ego* ordinarily more artful, more intelligent, and more clever than the individual'. [Alice Balint] The penis is regarded by the subject as at once himself and other than himself, because the functions of urination and later of erection are processes midway between the voluntary and involuntary, and because it is a capricious and as it were a foreign source of pleasure that is felt subjectively. The individual's specific transcendence takes concrete form in the penis and it is a source of pride. Because the phallus is thus set apart, man can bring into integration with his subjective individuality the life that overflows from it. It is easy to see, then, that the length of the penis, the force of the urinary jet, the strength of erection and ejaculation become for him the measure of his own worth . [I have been told of peasant children amusing themselves in excremental competition; the one who produced the most copious and solid faeces enjoyed a prestige unmatched by any other form of success, whether in games or even in fighting. The faecal mass here plays the same part as the penis – there is alienation in both cases.]

Thus the incarnation of transcendence in the phallus is a constant; and since it is also a constant for the child to feel himself transcended that is to say, frustrated in his own transcendence by the father – we therefore continually come upon the Freudian idea of the 'castration complex'. Not having that *alter ego,* the little girl is not alienated in a material thing and cannot retrieve her integrity. On this account she is led to make an object of her whole self, to set up herself as the Other. Whether she knows that she is or is not comparable with boys is secondary; the important point is that, even if she is unaware of it, the absence of the penis prevents her from being conscious of herself as a sexual being. From this flow many consequences. But the constants I have referred to do not for all that establish a fixed destiny – the phallus assumes such worth as it does because it symbolises a dominance that is exercised in other domains. If woman should succeed in establishing herself as subject, she would invent equivalents of the phallus; in fact, the doll, incarnating the promise of the baby that is to come in the future can become a possession more precious than the penis. There are matrilineal societies in which the women keep in their possession the *masks* in which the group finds alienation; in such societies the penis loses much of its glory. The fact is that a true human privilege is based upon the anatomical privilege only in virtue of the total situation. Psychoanalysis can establish its truths only in the historical context.

Woman can be defined by her consciousness of her own femininity no more satisfactorily than by saying that she is a female, for she acquires this consciousness under circumstances dependent upon the society of which she is a member. Interiorising the unconscious and the whole psychic life, the very language of psychoanalysis suggests that the drama of the individual unfolds within him – such words as *complex, tendency,* and so on make that implication. But a life is a relation to the world, and the individual defines himself by making his own choices through the world about him. We must therefore turn towards the world to find answers for the questions we are concerned with. In particular psychoanalysis fails to explain why woman is the *Other*. For Freud himself admits that the prestige of the penis is explained by the sovereignty of the father, and, as we have seen, he confesses that he is ignorant regarding the origin of male supremacy.

We therefore decline to accept the method of psychoanalysis, without rejecting *en bloc* the contributions of the science or denying the fertility of some of its insights. In the first place, we do not limit ourselves to regarding sexuality as something given. The insufficiency of this view is shown by the poverty of the resulting descriptions of the feminine libido; as I have already said, the psychoanalysts have never studied it directly, but only in taking the male libido as their point of departure. They seem to ignore the fundamental ambivalence of the attraction exerted on the female by the male. Freudians and Adlerians explain the anxiety felt by the female confronted by the masculine sex as being the inversion of a frustrated desire. Stekel saw more clearly that an original reaction was concerned, but he accounts for it in a superficial manner. Woman, he says, would fear decoration, penetration. pregnancy, and pain, and such fear would restrain her desire – but this explanation is too rational. Instead of holding that her desire is disguised in anxiety or is contested by fear, we should regard as an original fact this blending of urgency and apprehension which is female desire: it is the indissoluble synthesis of attraction and repulsion that characterises it. We may note that many female animals avoid copulation even as they are soliciting it, and we are tempted to accuse them of coquetry or hypocrisy; but it is absurd to pretend to explain primitive behaviour patterns by asserting their similarity to complex modes of conduct. On the contrary, the former are in truth at the source of the attitudes that in woman are called coquetry and hypocrisy. The notion of a 'passive libido' is baffling, since the libido has been defined, on the basis of the male, as a drive, an energy; but one would do no better to hold the opinion that a light could be at once yellow and blue – what is needed is the intuition of green. We would more fully encompass reality if instead of defining the libido in vague terms of 'energy' we brought the significance of sexuality into relation with that of other human attitudes – taking, capturing, eating, making, submitting, and so forth; for it is one of the various modes of apprehending an object. We should study also the qualities of the erotic object as it presents itself not only in the sexual act but also to observation in general. Such an investigation extends beyond the frame of psychoanalysis, which assumes eroticism as irreducible.

Furthermore, I shall pose the problem of feminine destiny quite otherwise: I shall place woman in a world of values and give her behaviour a dimension of liberty. I believe that she has the power to choose between the assertion of her transcendence and her alienation as object; she is not the plaything of contradictory drives; she devises solutions of diverse values in the ethical scale. Replacing value with authority, choice with drive, psychoanalysis offers an *Ersatz*, a substitute for morality – the concept of normality. This concept is certainly most useful in therapeutics, but it has spread through psychoanalysis in general to a disquieting extent. The descriptive schema is proposed as a law; and most assuredly a mechanistic psychology cannot accept the notion of moral invention; it can in strictness render an account of the *less* and never of the more; in strictness it can admit of checks, never of creations. If a subject does not show in his totality the development considered as normal, it will be said that his development has been arrested, and this arrest will be interpreted as a lack, a negation, but never as a positive decision. This it is, among other things, that makes the psychoanalysis of great men so shocking: we are told that such and such a transference, this or that sublimation, has not taken place in them; it is not suggested that perhaps they have refused to undergo the process, perhaps for good reasons of their own; it is not thought desirable to regard their behaviour as possibly motivated by purposes freely envisaged; the individual is always explained through ties with his past and not in respect to a future towards which he projects his aims. Thus the psychoanalysts never give us more than an inauthentic picture, and for the inauthentic there can hardly be found any other criterion than normality. Their statement of the feminine destiny is absolutely to the point in this connection. In the sense in which the psychoanalysts understand the term, 'to identify oneself' with the mother or with the father is *to alienate oneself* in a model, it is to prefer a foreign image to the spontaneous manifestation of one's own existence, it is to play at being. Woman is shown to us as enticed by two modes of alienation. Evidently to play at being a man will be for her a source of frustration; but to play at being a woman is also a delusion: to be a woman would mean to be the object, the *Other* – and the Other nevertheless remains subject in the midst of her resignation.

The true problem for woman is to reject these flights from reality and seek fulfilment in transcendence. The thing to do, then, is to see what possibilities are opened up for her through what are called the virile and the feminine attitudes. When a child takes the road indicated by one or the other of its parents, it may be because the child freely takes up their projects; its behaviour may be the result of a choice motivated by ends and aims. Even with Adler the will to power is only an absurd kind of energy; he denominates as 'masculine protest' every project involving transcendence. When a little girl climbs trees it is, according to Adler, just to show her equality with boys; it does not occur to him that she likes to climb trees. For the mother her child is something other than an 'equivalent of the penis'. To paint, to write, to engage in politics – these are not merely 'sublimations'; here we have aims that are willed for their own sakes. To deny it is to falsify all human history.

The Second Sex
by Simone de Beauvoir (1949)

Book One: Facts and Myths, Part I: Destiny

Chapter 3: The Point of View of Historical Materialism

THE theory of historical materialism has brought to light some most important truths. Humanity is not an animal species, it is a historical reality. Human society is an antiphysis – in a sense it is against nature; it does not passively submit to the presence of nature but rather takes over the control of nature on its own behalf. This arrogation is not an inward, subjective operation; it is accomplished objectively in practical action.

Thus woman could not be considered simply as a sexual organism, for among the biological traits, only those have importance that take on concrete value in action. Woman's awareness of herself is not defined exclusively by her sexuality: it reflects a situation that depends upon the economic organisation of society, which in turn indicates what stage of technical evolution mankind has attained. As we have seen, the two essential traits that characterise woman, biologically speaking, are the following: her grasp upon the world is less extended than man's, and she is more closely enslaved to the species.

But these facts take on quite different values according to the economic and social context. In human history grasp upon the world has never been defined by the naked body: the hand, with its opposable thumb, already anticipates the instrument that multiplies its power; from the most ancient records of prehistory, we see man always as armed. In times when heavy clubs were brandished and wild beasts held at bay, woman's physical weakness did constitute a glaring inferiority: if the instrument required strength slightly beyond that at woman's disposal, it was enough to make her appear utterly powerless. But, on the contrary, technique may annul the muscular inequality of man and woman: abundance makes for superiority only in the perspective of a need, and to have too much is no better than to have enough. Thus the control of many modern machines requires only a part of the masculine resources, and if the minimum demanded is not above the female's capacity, she becomes, as far as this work is concerned, man's equal. Today, of course, vast displays of energy can be controlled by pressing a button. As for the burdens of maternity, they assume widely varying importance according to the customs of the country: they are crushing if the woman is obliged to undergo frequent pregnancies and if she is compelled to nurse and raise the children without assistance; but if she procreates voluntarily and if society comes to her aid during pregnancy and is concerned with child welfare, the burdens of maternity are light and can be easily offset by suitable adjustments in working conditions.

Engels retraces the history of woman according to this perspective in *The Origin of the Family, Private Property, and the State*, showing that this history depended essentially on that of techniques. In the Stone Age, when the land belonged in common to all members of the clan, the rudimentary character of the primitive spade and hoe limited the possibilities of agriculture, so that woman's strength was adequate for gardening. In this primitive division of labour, the two sexes constituted in a way two classes, and there was equality between these classes. While man hunts and fishes, woman remains in the home; but the tasks of domesticity include productive labour – making pottery, weaving, gardening – and in consequence woman plays a large part in economic life. Through the discovery of copper, tin, bronze, and iron, and with the appearance of the plough, agriculture enlarges its scope, and intensive labour is called for in clearing woodland and cultivating the fields. Then man has recourse to the labour of other men, whom he reduces to slavery. Private property appears: master of slaves and of the earth, man becomes the proprietor also of woman. This was 'the great historical defeat of the feminine sex'. It is to be explained by the upsetting of the old division of labour which occurred in consequence of the invention of new tools. 'The same cause which had assured to woman the prime authority in the house – namely, her restriction to domestic duties – this same cause now assured the domination there of the man; for woman's housework henceforth sank into insignificance in comparison with man's productive labour – the latter as everything, the former a trifling auxiliary.' Then maternal authority gave place to paternal authority, property being inherited from father to son and no longer from woman to her clan. Here we see the emergence of the patriarchal family founded upon private property. In this type of family woman is subjugated. Man in his sovereignty indulges himself in sexual caprices, among others – he fornicates with slaves or courtesans or he practises polygamy. Wherever the local customs make reciprocity at all possible, the wife takes revenge through infidelity – marriage finds its natural fulfilment in adultery. This is woman's sole defence against the domestic slavery in which she is bound; and it is this economic oppression that gives rise to the social oppression to which she is subjected. Equality cannot be re-established until the two sexes enjoy equal rights in law; but this enfranchisement requires participation in general industry by the whole female sex. 'Woman can be emancipated only when she can take part on a large social scale in production and is engaged in domestic work only to an insignificant degree. And this has become possible only in the big industry of modern times, which not only admits of female labour on a grand scale but even formally demands it...'

Thus the fate of woman and that of socialism are intimately bound up together, as is shown also in Bebel's great work on woman. 'Woman and the proletariat,' he says, 'are both downtrodden.' Both are to be set free through the economic development consequent upon the social upheaval brought about by machinery. The problem of woman is reduced to the problem of her capacity for labour. Puissant at the time when techniques were suited to her capabilities, dethroned when she was no longer in a position to exploit them, woman regains in the modern world her equality with man. It is the resistance of the ancient capitalistic paternalism that in most countries prevents the concrete realisation of this equality; it will be realised on the day when this resistance is broken, as is the fact already in the Soviet Union, according to Soviet propaganda. And when the socialist society is established throughout the world, there will no longer be men and women, but only workers on a footing of equality.

Although this chain of thought as outlined by Engels marks an advance upon those we have been examining, we find it disappointing – the most important problems are slurred over. The turning-point of all history is the passage from the regime of community ownership to that of private property, and it is in no wise indicated how this could have come about. Engels himself declares in The *Origin of the Family* that 'at present we know nothing about it'; not only is he ignorant of the historical details: he does not even suggest any interpretation. Similarly, it is not clear that the institution of private property must necessarily have involved the enslavement of women. Historical materialism takes for granted facts that call for explanation: Engels assumes without discussion the bond of interest which ties man to property; but where does this interest, the source of social institutions, have its own source? Thus Engels's account remains superficial, and the truths that he does reveal are seemingly contingent, incidental. The fact is that we cannot plumb their meaning without going beyond the limits of historical materialism. It cannot provide solutions for the problems we have raised, because these concern the whole man and not that abstraction : *Homo oeconomicus*.

It would seem clear, for example, that the very concept of personal possession can be comprehensible only with reference to the original condition of the existent. For it to appear, there must have been at first an inclination in the subject to think of himself as basically individual, to assert the autonomy and separateness of his existence. We can see that this affirmation would have remained subjective, inward, without validity as long as the individual lacked the practical means for carrying it out objectively. Without adequate tools, he did not sense at first any power over the world, he felt lost in nature and in the group, passive, threatened, the plaything of obscure forces; he dared to think of himself only as identified with the clan: the totem, mana, the earth were group realities. The discovery of bronze enabled man, in the experience of hard and productive labour, to discover himself as creator; dominating nature, he was no longer afraid of it, and in the faceof obstacles overcome he found courage to see himself as an autonomous active force, to achieve self-fulfilment as an individual. [Gaston Bachelard in *La Terre et les réveries de fa volonté* makes among others a suggestive study of the blacksmith. He shows how man, through the hammer and the anvil, asserts himself and his individuality. 'The blacksmith's instant is an instant at once well marked off and magnified. It promotes the worker to the mastery of time, through the forcefulness of an instant' (p. 142); and farther on: 'The man at the forge accepts the challenge of the universe arrayed against him.']

But this accomplishment would never have been attained had not man originally willed it so; the lesson of work is not inscribed upon a passive subject: the subject shapes and masters himself in shaping and mastering the land.

On the other hand, the affirmation of the subject's individuality is not enough to explain property: each conscious individual through challenge, struggle, and single combat can endeavour to raise himself to sovereignty. For the challenge to have taken the form of *potlatch* or ceremonial exchange of gifts – that is, of an economic rivalry – and from this point on for first the chief and then the members of the clan to have laid claim to private property, required that there should be in man another original tendency. As we have seen in the preceding chapter, the existent succeeds in finding himself only in estrangement, in alienation; he seeks through the world to find himself in some shape, other than himself, which he makes his own. The clan encounters its own alienated existence in the totem, the mana, the terrain it occupies; and when the individual becomes distinguished from the community, he requires a personal incarnation. The mana becomes individualised in the chief, then in each individual; and at the same time each person tries to appropriate a piece of land, implements, crops. Man finds himself in these goods which are his because he has previously lost himself in them; and it is therefore understandable that he places upon them a value no less fundamental than upon his very life. Thus it is that man's interest in his property becomes an intelligible relation. But we see that this cannot be explained through the tool alone: we must grasp in its entirety the attitude of man wielding the tool, an attitude that implies an ontological substructure, a foundation in the nature of his being.

On the same grounds it is impossible to deduce the oppression of woman from the institution of private property. Here again the inadequacy of Engels's point of view is obvious. He saw clearly that woman's muscular weakness became a real point of inferiority only in its relation to the bronze and iron tool; but he did not see that the limitations of her capacity for labour constituted in themselves a concrete disadvantage only in a certain perspective. It is because man is a being of transcendence and ambition that he projects new urgencies through every new tool: when he had invented bronze implements, he was no longer content with gardens – he wanted to clear and cultivate vast fields. And it was not from the bronze itself that this desire welled up. Woman's incapacity brought about her ruin because man regarded her in the perspective of his project for enrichment and expansion. And this project is still not enough to explain why she was oppressed; for the division of labour between the sexes could have meant a friendly association. If the original relation between a man and his fellows was exclusively a relation of friendship, we could not account for any type of enslavement; but no, this phenomenon is a result of the imperialism of the human consciousness, seeking always to exercise its sovereignty in objective fashion. If the human consciousness had not included the original category of the Other and an original aspiration to dominate the Other, the invention of the bronze tool could not have caused the oppression of woman.

No more does Engels account for the peculiar nature of this oppression. He tried to reduce the antagonism of the sexes to class conflict, but he was half-hearted in the attempt; the thesis is simply untenable. It is true that division of labour according to sex and the consequent oppression bring to mind in some ways the division of society by classes, but it is impossible to confuse the two. For one thing, there is no biological basis for the separation of classes. Again, the slave in his toil is conscious of himself as opposed to his master; and the proletariat has always put its condition to the test in revolt, thereby going back to essentials and constituting a threat to its exploiters. And what it has aimed at is its own disappearance as a class. I have pointed out in the Introduction how different woman's situation is, particularly on account of the community of life and interests which entails her solidarity with man, and also because he finds in her an accomplice; no desire for revolution dwells within her, nor any thought of her own disappearance as a sex – all she asks is that certain sequels of sexual differentiation be abolished.

What is still more serious, woman cannot in good faith be regarded simply as a worker; for her reproductive function is as important as her productive capacity, no less in the social economy than in the individual life. In some periods, indeed, it is more useful to produce offspring than to plough the soil. Engels slighted the problem, simply remarking that the socialist community would abolish the family – certainly an abstract solution. We know how often and how radically Soviet Russia has had to change its policy on the family according to the varying relation between the immediate needs of production and those of re-population. But for that matter, to do away with the family is not necessarily to emancipate woman. Such examples as Sparta and the Nazi regime prove that she can be none the less oppressed by the males, for all her direct attachment to the State.

A truly socialist ethics, concerned to uphold justice without suppressing liberty and to impose duties upon individuals without abolishing individuality, will find most embarrassing the problems posed by the condition of woman. It is impossible simply to equate gestation with a *task,* a piece of work, or with a service, such as military service. Woman's life is more seriously broken in upon by a demand for children than by regulation of the citizen's employment – no state has ever ventured to establish obligatory copulation. In the sexual act and in maternity not only time and strength but also essential values are involved for woman. Rationalist materialism tries in vain to disregard this dramatic aspect of sexuality; for it is impossible to bring the sexual instinct under a code of regulations. Indeed, as Freud said, it is not sure that it does not bear within itself a denial of its own satisfaction. What is certain is that it does not permit of integration with the social, because there is in eroticism a revolt of the instant against time, of the individual against the universal. In proposing to direct and exploit it, there is risk of killing it, for it is impossible to deal at will with living spontaneity as one deals at will with inert matter; and no more can it be obtained by force, as a privilege may be.

There is no way of directly compelling woman to bring forth: all that can be done is to put her in a situation where maternity is for her the sole outcome – the law or the mores enjoin marriage, birth control and abortion are prohibited, divorce is forbidden. These ancient patriarchal restraints are just what Soviet Russia has brought back today; Russia has revived the paternalistic concepts of marriage. And in doing so, she has been induced to ask woman once more to make of herself an erotic object: in a recent pronouncement female Soviet citizens were requested to pay careful attention to their garb, to use make-up, to employ the arts of coquetry in holding their husbands and fanning the flame of desire. As this case shows clearly, it is impossible to regard woman simply as a productive force: she is for man a sexual partner, a reproducer, an erotic object – an Other through whom he seeks himself. In vain have the totalitarian or authoritative regimes with one accord prohibited psychoanalysis and declared that individual, personal drama is out of order for citizens loyally integrated with the community; the erotic experience remains one in which generality is always regained by an individuality. And for a democratic socialism in which classes are abolished but not individuals, the question of individual destiny would keep all its importance – and hence sexual differentiation would keep all its importance. The sexual relation that joins woman to man is not the same as that which he bears to her; and the bond that unites her to the child is *sui generis*, unique. She was not created by the bronze tool alone; and the machine tool alone will not abolish her. To claim for her every right, every chance to be an all-round human being does not mean that we should be blind to her peculiar situation. And in order to comprehend we must look beyond the historical materialism that man and woman no more than economic units.

So it is that we reject for the same reasons both the sexual monism of Freud and the economic monism of Engels. A psychoanalyst will interpret the claims of woman as phenomena of the 'masculine protest'; for the Marxist, on the contrary, her sexuality only expresses her economic situation in more or less complex, roundabout fashion. But the categories of 'clitorid' and 'vaginal', like the categories of 'bourgeois' or 'proletarian', are equally inadequate to encompass a concrete woman. Underlying all individual drama, as it underlies the economic history of mankind, there is an existentialist foundation that alone enables us to understand in its unity that particular form of being which we call a human life. The virtue of Freudianism derives from the fact that the existent is a body: what he experiences as a body confronted by other bodies expresses his existential situation concretely. Similarly, what is true in the Marxian thesis is that the ontological aspirations – the projects for becoming – of the existent take concrete form according to the material possibilities offered, especially those opened up by technological advances. But unless they are integrated into the totality of human reality, sexuality and technology alone can explain nothing. That is why in Freud the prohibitions of the super-ego and the drives of the ego appear to be contingent, and why in Engels's account of the history of the family the most important developments seem to arise according to the caprices of mysterious fortune. In our attempt to discover woman we shall not reject certain contributions of biology, of psychoanalysis, and of historical materialism; but we shall hold that the body, the sexual life, and the resources of technology exist concretely for man only in so far as he grasps them in the total perspective of his existence. The value of muscular strength, of the phallus, of the tool can be defined only in a world of values; it is determined by the basic project through which the existent seeks transcendence.

From Part II of *The Second Sex*. Simone de Beauvoir 1949

On the Master-Slave Relation

Certain passages in the argument employed by Hegel in defining the relation of master to slave apply much better to the relation of man to woman. The advantage of the master, he says, comes from his affirmation of Spirit as against Life through the fact that he risks his own life; but in fact the conquered slave has known this same risk. Whereas woman is basically an existent who gives Life and does not risk *her* life, between her and the male there has been no combat. Hegel's definition would seem to apply especially well to her. He says: 'The other consciousness is the dependent consciousness for whom the essential reality is the animal type of life; that is to say, a mode of living bestowed by another entity.' But this relation is to be distinguished from the relation of subjugation because woman also aspires to and recognizes the values that are concretely attained by the male. He it is who opens up the future to which she also reaches out. In truth women have never set up female values in opposition to male values; it is man who, desirous of maintaining masculine prerogatives, has invented that divergence. Men have presumed to create a feminine domain – the kingdom of life, of immanence – only in order to lock up women therein. But it is regardless of sex that the existent seeks self-justification through transcendence – the very submission of women is proof of that statement. What they demand today is to be recognized as existents by the same right as men and not to subordinate existence to life, the human being to its animality.

An existentialist perspective has enabled us, then, to understand how the biological and economic condition of the primitive horde must have led to male supremacy. The female, to a greater extent than the male, is the prey of the species; and the human race has always sought to escape its specific destiny. The support of life became for man an activity and a project through the invention of the tool; but in maternity woman remained closely bound to her body, like an animal. It is because humanity calls itself in question in the matter of living – that is to say, values the reasons for living above mere life – that, confronting woman, man assumes mastery. Man's design is not to repeat himself in time: it is to take control of the instant and mould the future. It is male activity that in creating values has made of existence itself a value; this activity has prevailed over the confused forces of life; it has subdued Nature and Woman. We must now see how this situation has been perpetuated and how it has evolved through the ages. What place has humanity made for this portion of itself which, while included within it, is defined as the Other? What rights have been conceded to it? How have men defined it?

The Second Sex
by Simone de Beauvoir (1949)

Conclusion

'NO, WOMAN is not our brother; through indolence and deceit we have made of her a being apart, unknown, having no weapon other than her sex, which not only means constant warfare but unfair warfare – adoring or hating, but never a straight friend, a being in a legion with *esprit de corps* and freemasonry – the defiant gestures of the eternal little slave.'

Many men would still subscribe to these words of Laforgue; many think that there will always be 'strife and dispute', as Montaigne put it, and that fraternity will never be possible. The fact is that today neither men nor women are satisfied with each other. But the question is to know whether there is an original curse that condemns them to rend each other or whether the conflicts in which they are opposed merely mark a transitional moment in human history.

Legends notwithstanding, no physiological destiny imposes an eternal hostility upon Male and Female as such; even the famous praying mantis devours her male only for want of other food and for the good of the species: it is to this, the species, that all individuals are subordinated, from the top to the bottom of the scale of animal life. Moreover, humanity is something more than a mere species: it is a historical development; it is to be defined by the manner in which it deals with its natural, fixed characteristics, its facticité. Indeed, even with the most extreme bad faith, it is impossible to demonstrate the existence of a rivalry between the human male and female of a truly physiological nature. Further, their hostility may be allocated rather to that intermediate terrain between biology and psychology: psychoanalysis. Woman, we are told, envies man his penis and wishes to castrate him; but the childish desire for the penis is important in the life of the adult woman only if she feels her femininity as a mutilation; and then it is as a symbol of all the privileges of manhood that she wishes to appropriate the male organ. We may readily agree that her dream of castration has this symbolic significance: she wishes, it is thought, to deprive the male of his transcendence.

But her desire, as we have seen, is much more ambiguous: she wishes, in a contradictory fashion, *to have* this transcendence, which is to suppose that she at once respects it and denies it, that she intends at once to throw herself into it and keep it within herself. This is to say that the drama does not unfold on a sexual level; further, sexuality has never seemed to us to define a destiny, to furnish in itself the key to human behaviour, but to express the totality of a situation that it only helps to define. The battle of the sexes is not implicit in the anatomy of man and woman. The truth is that when one evokes it, one takes for granted that in the timeless realm of Ideas a battle is being waged between those vague essences the Eternal Feminine and the Eternal Masculine; and one neglects the fact that this titanic combat assumes on earth two totally different forms, corresponding with two different moments of history.

The woman who is shut up in immanence endeavours to hold man in that prison also; thus the prison will become interchangeable with the world, and woman will no longer suffer from being confined there: mother, wife, sweetheart are the jailers. Society, being codified by man, decrees that woman is inferior: she can do away with this inferiority only by destroying the male's superiority. She sets about mutilating, dominating man, she contradicts him, she denies his truth and his values. But in doing this she is only defending herself; it was neither a changeless essence nor a mistaken choice that doomed her to immanence, to inferiority. They were imposed upon her. All oppression creates a state of war. And this is no exception. The existent who is regarded as inessential cannot fail to demand the re-establishment of her sovereignty.

Today the combat takes a different shape; instead of wishing to put man in a prison, woman endeavours to escape from one; she no longer seeks to drag him into the realms of immanence but to emerge, herself, into the light of transcendence. Now the attitude of the males creates a new conflict: it is with a bad grace that the man lets her go. He is very well pleased to remain the sovereign subject, the absolute superior, the essential being; he refuses to accept his companion as an equal in any concrete way. She replies to his lack of confidence in her by assuming an aggressive attitude. It is no longer a question of a war between individuals each shut up in his or her sphere: a caste claiming its rights attacks and is resisted by the privileged caste. Here two transcendences are face to face; instead of displaying mutual recognition, each free being wishes to dominate the other.

This difference of attitude is manifest on the sexual plane as on the spiritual plane. The 'feminine' woman in making herself prey tries to reduce man, also, to her carnal passivity; she occupies herself in catching him in her trap, in enchaining him by means of the desire she arouses in him in submissively making herself a thing. The emancipated woman, on the contrary, wants to be active, a taker, and refuses the passivity man means to impose on her. The 'modern' woman accepts masculine values: she prides herself on thinking, taking action, working, creating, on the same terms as men; instead of seeking to disparage them, she declares herself their equal.

In so far as she expresses herself in definite action, this claim is legitimate, and male insolence must then bear the blame. But in men's defence it must be said that women are wont to confuse the issue. Many women, in order to show by their successes their equivalence to men, try to secure male support by sexual means; they play on both sides, demanding old-fashioned respect and modern esteem, banking on their old magic and their new rights. It is understandable that a man becomes irritated and puts himself on the defensive; but he is also double-dealing when he requires woman to play the game fairly while he denies her the indispensable trump cards through distrust and hostility. Indeed, the struggle cannot be clearly drawn between them, since woman is opaque in her very being; she stands before man not as a subject but as an object paradoxically endued with subjectivity; she takes herself simultaneously *as self* and *as other*, a contradiction that entails baffling consequences. When she makes weapons at once of her weakness and of her strength, it is not a matter of designing calculation: she seeks salvation spontaneously in the way that has been imposed on her, that of passivity, at the same time when she is actively demanding her sovereignty; and no doubt this procedure is unfair tactics, but it is dictated by the ambiguous situation assigned her. Man, however, becomes indignant when he treats her as a free and independent being and then realises that she is still a trap for him; if he gratifies and satisfies her in her posture as prey, he finds her claims to autonomy irritating; whatever he does, he feels tricked and she feels wronged.

The quarrel will go on as long as men and women fail to recognise each other as equals; that is to say, as long as femininity is perpetuated as such. Which sex is the more eager to maintain it? Woman, who is being emancipated from it, wishes none the less to retain its privileges; and man, in that case, wants her to assume its limitations. 'It is easier to accuse one sex than to excuse the other,' says Montaigne. It is vain to apportion praise and blame. The truth is that if the vicious circle is so hard to break, it is because the two sexes are each the victim at once of the other and of itself. Between two adversaries confronting each other in their pure liberty, an agreement could be easily reached: the more so as the war profits neither. But the complexity of the whole affair derives from the fact that each camp is giving aid and comfort to the enemy; woman is pursuing a dream of submission, man a dream of identification. Want of authenticity does not pay: each blames the other for the unhappiness he or she has incurred in yielding to the temptations of the easy way; what man and woman loathe in each other is the shattering frustration of each one's own bad faith and baseness.

We have seen why men enslaved women in the first place; the devaluation of femininity has been a necessary step in human evolution, but it might have led to collaboration between the two sexes; oppression is to be explained by the tendency of the existent to flee from himself by means of identification with the other, whom he oppresses to that end. In each individual man that tendency exists today; and the vast majority yield to it. The husband wants to find himself in his wife, the lover in his mistress, in the form of a stone image; he is seeking in her the myth of his virility, of his sovereignty, of his immediate reality. But he is himself the slave of his double: what an effort to build up an image in which he is always in danger! In spite of everything his success in this depends upon the capricious freedom of women: he must constantly try to keep this propitious to him. Man is concerned with the effort to appear male, important, superior; he pretends so as to get pretence in return; he, too, is aggressive, uneasy; he feels hostility for women because he is afraid of them, he is afraid of them because he is afraid of the personage, the image, with which he identifies himself. What time and strength he squanders in liquidating, sublimating, transferring complexes, in talking about women, in seducing them, in fearing them! He would be liberated himself in their liberation. But this is precisely what he dreads. And so he obstinately persists in the mystifications intended to keep woman in her chains.

That she is being tricked, many men have realised. 'What a misfortune to be a woman! And yet the misfortune, when one is a woman, is at bottom not to comprehend that it is one,' says Kierkegaard. [In *Vino Veritas*. He says further: 'Politeness is pleasing – essentially – to woman, and the fact that she accepts it without hesitation is explained by nature's care for the weaker, for the unfavoured being, and for one to whom an illusion means more than a material compensation. But this illusion, precisely, is fatal to her ... To feel oneself freed from distress thanks to something imaginary, to be the dupe of something imaginary, is that not a still deeper mockery? ... Woman is very far from being *verwahrlost* (neglected), but in another sense she is, since she can never free herself from the illusion that nature has used to console her.'] For a long time there have been efforts to disguise this misfortune. For example, guardianship has been done away with: women have been given 'protectors', and if they are invested with the rights of the old-time guardians, it is in woman's own interest. To forbid her working, to keep her at home, is to defend her against herself and to assure her happiness. We have seen what poetic veils are thrown over her monotonous burdens of housekeeping and maternity: in exchange for her liberty she has received the false treasures of her 'femininity'. Balzac illustrates this manoeuvre very well in counselling man to treat her as a slave while persuading her that she is a queen. Less cynical, many men try to convince themselves that she is really privileged. There are American sociologists who seriously teach today the theory of 'low-class gain', that is to say, the benefits enjoyed by the lower orders. In France, also, it has often been proclaimed – although in a less scientific manner – that the workers are very fortunate in not being obliged to 'keep up appearances'. Like the carefree wretches gaily scratching at their vermin, like the merry Negroes laughing under the lash, and those joyous Tunisian Arabs burying their starved children with a smile, woman enjoys that incomparable privilege: irresponsibility. Free from troublesome burdens and cares, she obviously has 'the better part'. But it is disturbing that with an obstinate perversity – connected no doubt with original sin – down through the centuries and in all countries, the people who have the better part are always crying to their benefactors: 'It is too much! I will be satisfied with yours!' But the munificent capitalists, the generous colonists, the superb males, stick to their guns: 'Keep the better part, hold on to it!'

It must be admitted that the males find in woman more complicity than the oppressor usually finds in the oppressed. And in bad faith they take authorisation from this to declare that she has desired the destiny they have imposed on her. We have seen that all the main features of her training combine to bar her from the roads of revolt and adventure. Society in general – beginning with her respected parents – lies to her by praising the lofty values of love, devotion, the gift of herself, and then concealing from her the fact that neither lover nor husband nor yet her children will be inclined to accept the burdensome charge of all that. She cheerfully believes these lies because they invite her to follow the easy slope: in this others commit their worst crime against her; throughout her life from childhood on, they damage and corrupt her by designating as her true vocation this submission, which is the temptation of every existent in the anxiety of liberty. If a child is taught idleness by being amused all day long and never being led to study, or shown its usefulness, it will hardly be said, when he grows up, that he chose to be incapable and ignorant; yet this is how woman is brought up, without ever being impressed with the necessity of taking charge of her own existence. So she readily lets herself come to count on the protection, love, assistance, and supervision of others, she lets herself be fascinated with the hope of self-realisation without doing anything. She does wrong in yielding to the temptation; but man is in no position to blame her, since he has led her into the temptation. When conflict arises between them, each will hold the other responsible for the situation; she will reproach him with having made her what she is: 'No one taught me to reason or to earn my own living'; he will reproach her with having accepted the consequences: 'You don't know anything you are an incompetent,' and so on. Each sex thinks it can justify itself by taking the offensive; but the wrongs done by one do not make the other innocent.

The innumerable conflicts that set men and women against one another come from the fact that neither is prepared to assume all the consequences of this situation which the one has offered and the other accepted. The doubtful concept of 'equality in inequality', which the one uses to mask his despotism and the other to mask her cowardice, does not stand the test of experience: in their exchanges, woman appeals to the theoretical equality she has been guaranteed, and man the concrete inequality that exists. The result is that in every association an endless debate goes on concerning the ambiguous meaning of the words give and take: she complains of giving her all, he protests that she takes his all. Woman has to learn that exchanges – it is a fundamental law of political economy – are based on the value the merchandise offered has for the buyer, and not for the seller: she has been deceived in being persuaded that her worth is priceless. The truth is that for man she is an amusement, a pleasure, company, an inessential boon; he is for her the meaning, the justification of her existence. The exchange, therefore, is not of two items of equal value.

This inequality will be especially brought out in the fact that the time they spend together – which fallaciously seems to be the same time – does not have the same value for both partners. During the evening the lover spends with his mistress he could be doing something of advantage to his career, seeing friends, cultivating business relationships, seeking recreation; for a man normally integrated in society, time is a positive value: money, reputation, pleasure. For the idle, bored woman, on the contrary, it is a burden she wishes to get rid of; when she succeeds in killing time, it is a benefit to her: the man's presence is pure profit. In a liaison what most clearly interests the man, in many cases, is the sexual benefit he gets from it: if need be, he can be content to spend no more time with his mistress than is required for the sexual act; but – with exceptions – what she, on her part, wants is to kill all the excess time she has on her hands; and – like the greengrocer who will not sell potatoes unless the customer will take turnips also – she will not yield her body unless her lover will take hours of conversation and 'going out' into the bargain. A balance is reached if, on the whole, the cost does not seem too high to the man, and this depends, of course, on the strength of his desire and the importance he gives to what is to be sacrificed. But if the woman demands – offers – too much time, she becomes wholly intrusive, like the river overflowing its banks, and the man will prefer to have nothing rather than too much. Then she reduces her demands; but very often the balance is reached at the cost of a double tension: she feels that the man has 'had' her at a bargain, and he thinks her price is too high. This analysis, of course, is put in somewhat humorous terms; but – except for those affairs of jealous and exclusive passion in which the man wants total possession of the woman – this conflict constantly appears in cases of affection, desire, and even love. He always has 'other things to do' with his time; whereas she has time to kill; and he considers much of the time she gives him not as a gift but as a burden.

As a rule he consents to assume the burden because he knows very well that he is on the privileged side, he has a bad conscience; and if he is of reasonable good will he tries to compensate for the inequality by being generous. He prides himself on his compassion, however, and at the first clash he treats the woman as ungrateful and thinks, with some irritation: 'I'm too good for her.' She feels she is behaving like a beggar when she is convinced of the high value of her gifts, and that humiliates her.

Here we find the explanation of the cruelty that woman often shows she is capable of practising; she has a good conscience because she is on the unprivileged side; she feels she is under no obligation to deal gently with the favoured caste, and her only thought is to defend herself. She will even be very happy if she has occasion to show her resentment to a lover who has not been able to satisfy all her demands: since he does not give her enough, she takes savage delight in taking back everything from him. At this point the wounded lover suddenly discovers the value *in toto* of a liaison each moment of which he held more or less in contempt: he is ready to promise her everything, even though he will feel exploited again when he has to make good. He accuses his mistress of blackmailing him: she calls him stingy; both feel wronged.

Once again it is useless to apportion blame and excuses: justice can never be done in the midst of injustice. A colonial administrator has no possibility of acting rightly towards the natives, nor a general towards his soldiers; the only solution is to be neither colonist nor military chief; but a man could not prevent himself from being a man. So there he is, culpable in spite of himself and labouring under the effects of a fault he did not himself commit; and here she is, victim and shrew in spite of herself. Sometimes he rebels and becomes cruel, but then he makes himself an accomplice of the injustice, and the fault becomes really his. Sometimes he lets himself be annihilated, devoured, by his demanding victim; but in that case he feels duped. Often he stops at a compromise that at once belittles him and leaves him ill at ease. A well-disposed man will be more tortured by the situation than the woman herself: in a sense it is always better to be on the side of the vanquished; but if she is well-disposed also, incapable of self-sufficiency, reluctant to crush the man with the weight of her destiny, she struggles in hopeless confusion.

In daily life we meet with an abundance of these cases which are incapable of satisfactory solution because they are determined by unsatisfactory conditions. A man who is compelled to go on materially and morally supporting a woman whom he no longer loves feels he is victimised; but if he abandons without resources the woman who has pledged her whole life to him, she will be quite as unjustly victimised. The evil originates not in the perversity of individuals and bad faith first appears when each blames the other – it originates rather in a situation against which all individual action is powerless. Women are 'clinging', they are a dead weight, and they suffer for it; the point is that their situation is like that of a parasite sucking out the living strength of another organism. Let them be provided with living strength of their own, let them have the means to attack the world and wrest from it their own subsistence, and their dependence will be abolished – that of man also. There is no doubt that both men and women will profit greatly from the new situation.

A world where men and women would be equal is easy to visualise, for that precisely is what the Soviet Revolution *promised*: women reared and trained exactly like men were to work under the same conditions [That certain too laborious occupations were to be closed to women is not in contradiction to this project. Even among men there is an increasing effort to obtain adaptation to profession; their varying physical and mental capacities limit their possibilities of choice; what is asked is that, in any case, no line of sex or caste be drawn.] and for the same wages. Erotic liberty was to be recognised by custom, but the sexual act was not to be considered a 'service' to be paid for; woman was to be obliged to provide herself with other ways of earning a living; marriage was to be based on a free agreement that the contracting parties could break at will; maternity was to be voluntary, which meant that contraception and abortion were to be authorised and that, on the other hand, all mothers and their children were to have exactly the same rights, in or out of marriage; pregnancy leaves were to be paid for by the State, which would assume charge of the children, signifying not that they would be taken away from their parents, but that they would not be abandoned to them.

But is it enough to change laws, institutions, customs, public opinion, and the whole social context, for men and women to become truly equal? 'Women will always be women,' say the sceptics. Other seers prophesy that in casting off their femininity they will not succeed in changing themselves into men and they will become monsters. This would be to admit that the woman of today is a creation of nature; it must be repeated once more that in human society nothing is natural and that woman, like much else, is a product elaborated by civilisation. The intervention of others in her destiny is fundamental: if this action took a different direction, it would produce a quite different result. Woman is determined not by her hormones or by mysterious instincts, but by the manner in which her body and her relation to the world are modified through the action of others than herself. The abyss that separates the adolescent boy and girl has been deliberately widened between them since earliest childhood; later on, woman could not be other than what she *was made,* and that past was bound to shadow her for life. If we appreciate its influence, we see dearly that her destiny is not predetermined for all eternity.

We must not believe, certainly, that a change in woman's economic condition alone is enough to transform her, though this factor has been and remains the basic factor in her evolution; but until it has brought about the moral, social, cultural, and other consequences that it promises and requires, the new woman cannot appear. At this moment they have been realised nowhere, in Russia no more than in France or the United States; and this explains why the woman of today is torn between the past and the future. She appears most often as a 'true woman' disguised as a man, and she feels herself as ill at ease in her flesh as in her masculine garb. She must shed her old skin and cut her own new clothes. This she could do only through a social evolution. No single educator could fashion a *female human being* today who would be the exact homologue of the *male human being*; if she is brought up like a boy, the young girl feels she *is* an oddity and thereby she is given a new kind of sex specification. Stendhal understood this when he said: 'The forest must be planted all at once.' But if we imagine, on the contrary, a society in which the equality of the sexes would be concretely realised, this equality would find new expression in each individual.

If the little girl were brought up from the first with the same demands and rewards, the same severity and the same freedom, as her brothers, taking part in the same studies, the same games, promised the same future, surrounded with women and men who seemed to her undoubted equals, the meanings of the castration complex and of the Oedipus complex would be profoundly modified. Assuming on the same basis as the father the material and moral responsibility of the couple, the mother would enjoy the same lasting prestige; the child would perceive around her an androgynous world and not a masculine world. Were she emotionally more attracted to her father – which is not even sure – her love for him would be tinged with a will to emulation and not a feeling of powerlessness; she would not be oriented towards passivity. Authorised to test her powers in work and sports, competing actively with the boys, she would not find the absence of the penis – compensated by the promise of a child enough to give rise to an inferiority complex; correlatively the boy would not have a superiority complex if it were not instilled into him and if he looked up to women with as much respect as to men. [I knew a little boy of eight who lived with his mother, aunt and grandmother, all independent and active women, and his weak old half-crippled grandfather. He had a crushing inferiority complex in regard to the feminine sex, although he made efforts to combat it. At school he scorned comrades and teachers because they were miserable males.] The little girl would not seek sterile compensation in narcissism and dreaming, she would not take her fate for granted; she would be interested in what she was doing, she would throw herself without reserve into undertakings.

I have already pointed out how much easier the transformation of puberty would be if she looked beyond it, like the boys, towards a free adult future: menstruation horrifies her only because it is an abrupt descent into femininity. She would also take her young eroticism in much more tranquil fashion if she did not feel a frightened disgust for her destiny as a whole, coherent sexual information would do much to help her over this crisis. And thanks to coeducational schooling, the august mystery of Man would have no occasion to enter her mind: it would be eliminated by everyday familiarity and open rivalry.

Objections raised against this system always imply respect for sexual taboos; but the effort to inhibit all sex curiosity and pleasure in the child is quite useless; one succeeds only in creating repressions, obsessions, neuroses. The excessive sentimentality, homosexual fervours, and platonic crushes of adolescent girls, with all their train of silliness and frivolity, are much more injurious than a little childish sex play and a few definite sex experiences. It would be beneficial above all for the young girl not to be influenced against taking charge herself of her own existence, for then she would not seek a demigod in the male – merely a comrade, a friend, a partner. Eroticism and love would take on the nature of free transcendence and not that of resignation; she could experience them as a relation between equals. There is no intention, of course, to remove by a stroke of the pen all the difficulties that the child has to overcome in changing into an adult; the most intelligent, the most tolerant education could not relieve the child of experiencing things for herself; what could be asked is that obstacles should not be piled gratuitously in her path. Progress is already shown by the fact that 'vicious' little girls are no longer cauterised with a red-hot iron. Psychoanalysis has given parents some instruction, but the conditions under which, at the present time, the sexual training and initiation of woman are accomplished are so deplorable that none of the objections advanced against the idea of a radical change could be considered valid. It is not a question of abolishing in woman the contingencies and miseries of the human condition, but of giving her the means for transcending them.

Woman is the victim of no mysterious fatality; the peculiarities that identify her as specifically a woman get their importance from the significance placed upon them. They can be surmounted, in the future, when they are regarded in new perspectives. Thus, as we have seen, through her erotic experience woman feels – and often detests – the domination of the male; but this is no reason to conclude that her ovaries condemn her to live for ever on her knees. Virile aggressiveness seems like a lordly privilege only within a system that in its entirety conspires to affirm masculine sovereignty; and woman *feels* herself profoundly passive in the sexual act only because she already thinks of herself as such. Many modern women who lay claim to their dignity as human beings still envisage their erotic life from the standpoint of a tradition of slavery: since it seems to them humiliating to lie beneath the man, to be penetrated by him, they grow tense in frigidity. But if the reality were different, the meaning expressed symbolically in amorous gestures and postures would be different, too: a woman who pays and dominates her lover can, for example, take pride in her superb idleness and consider that she is enslaving the male who is actively exerting himself. And here and now there are many sexually well-balanced couples whose notions of victory and defeat are giving place to the idea of an exchange.

As a matter of fact, man, like woman, is flesh, therefore passive, the plaything of his hormones and of the species, the restless prey of his desires. And she, like him, in the midst of the carnal fever, is a consenting, a voluntary gift, an activity; they live out in their several fashions the strange ambiguity of existence made body. In those combats where they think they confront one another, it is really against the self that each one struggles, projecting into the partner that part of the self which is repudiated; instead of living out the ambiguities of their situation, each tries to make the other bear the objection and tries to reserve the honour for the self. If, however, both should assume the ambiguity with. a clear-sighted modesty, correlative of an authentic pride, they would see each other as equals and would live out their erotic drama in amity. The fact that we are human beings is infinitely more important than all the peculiarities that distinguish human beings from one another; it is never the given that confers superiorities: 'virtue', as the ancients called it, is defined at the level of 'that which depends on us'. In both sexes is played out the same drama of the flesh and the spirit, of finitude and transcendence; both are gnawed away by time and laid in wait for by death, they have the same essential need for one another; and they can gain from their liberty the same glory. If they were to taste it, they would no longer be tempted to dispute fallacious privileges, and fraternity between them could then come into existence.

I shall be told that all this is utopian fancy, because woman cannot be transformed unless society has first made her really the equal of man. Conservatives have never failed in such circumstances to refer to that vicious circle; history, however, does not revolve. If a caste is kept in a state of inferiority, no doubt it remains inferior; but liberty can break the circle. Let the Negroes vote and they become worthy of having the vote; let woman be given responsibilities and she is able to assume them. The fact is that oppressors cannot be expected to make a move of gratuitous generosity; but at one time the revolt of the oppressed, at another time even the very evolution of the privileged caste itself, creates new situations; thus men have been led, in their own interest, to give partial emancipation to women: it remains only for women to continue their ascent, and the successes they are obtaining are an encouragement for them to do so. It seems almost certain that sooner or later they will arrive at complete economic and social equality, which will bring about an inner metamorphosis.

However this may be, there will be some to object that if such a world is possible it is not desirable. When woman is 'the same' as her male, life will lose its salt and spice. This argument, also, has lost its novelty: those interested in perpetuating present conditions are always in tears about the marvellous past that is about to disappear, without having so much as a smile for the young future. It is quite true that doing away with the slave trade meant death to the great plantations, magnificent with azaleas and camellias, it meant ruin to the whole refined Southern civilisation. In the attics of time rare old laces have joined the clear pure voices of the Sistine *castrati,* and there is a certain 'feminine charm' that is also on the way to the same dusty repository. I agree that he would be a barbarian indeed who failed to appreciate exquisite flowers, rare lace, the crystal-clear voice of the eunuch, and feminine charm.

When the 'charming woman' shows herself in all her splendour, she is a much more exalting object than the 'idiotic paintings, over-doors, scenery, showman's garish signs, popular reproductions', that excited Rimbaud; adorned with the most modern artifices, beautified according to the newest techniques, she comes down from the remoteness of the ages, from Thebes, from Crete, from Chichén-Itzá; and she is also the totem set up deep in the African jungle; she is a helicopter and she is a bird; and there is this, the greatest wonder of all: under her tinted hair the forest murmur becomes a thought, and words issue from her breasts. Men stretch forth avid hands towards the marvel, but when they grasp it it is gone; the wife, the mistress, speak like everybody else through their mouths: their words are worth just what they are worth; their breasts also. Does such a fugitive miracle – and one so rare – justify us in perpetuating a situation that is baneful for both sexes? One can appreciate the beauty of flowers, the charm of women, and appreciate them at their true value; if these treasures cost blood or misery, they must be sacrificed.

But in truth this sacrifice seems to men a peculiarly heavy one; few of them really wish in their hearts for woman to succeed in making it; those among them who hold woman in contempt see in the sacrifice nothing for them to gain, those who cherish her see too much that they would lose. And it is true that the evolution now in progress threatens more than feminine charm alone: in beginning to exist for herself, woman will relinquish the function as double and mediator to which she owes her privileged place in the masculine universe; to man, caught between the silence of nature and the demanding presence of other free beings, a creature who is at once his like and a passive thing seems a great treasure. The guise in which he conceives his companion may be mythical, but the experiences for which she is the source or the pretext are none the less real: there are hardly any more precious, more intimate, more ardent. There is no denying that feminine dependence, inferiority, woe, give women their special character; assuredly woman's autonomy, if it spares men many troubles, will also deny them many conveniences; assuredly there are certain forms of the sexual adventure which will be lost in the world of tomorrow. But this does not mean that love, happiness, poetry, dream, will be banished from it.

Let us not forget that our lack of imagination always depopulates the future; for us it is only an abstraction; each one of us secretly deplores the absence there of the one who was himself. But the humanity of tomorrow will be living in its flesh and in its conscious liberty; that time will be its present and it will in turn prefer it. New relations of flesh and sentiment of which we have no conception will arise between the sexes; already, indeed, there have appeared between men and women friendships, rivalries, complicities, comradeships – chaste or sensual – which past centuries could not have conceived. To mention one point, nothing could seem more debatable than the opinion that dooms the new world to uniformity and hence to boredom. I fail to see that this present world is free from boredom or that liberty ever creates uniformity.

To begin with, there will always be certain differences between man and woman; her eroticism, and therefore her sexual world, have a special form of their own and therefore cannot fail to engender a sensuality, a sensitivity, of a special nature. This means that her relations to her own body, to that of the male, to the child, will never be identical with those the male bears to his own body, to that of the female, and to the child; those who make much of 'equality in difference' could not with good grace refuse to grant me the possible existence of differences in equality. Then again, it is institutions that create uniformity. Young and pretty, the slaves of the harem are always the same in the sultan's embrace; Christianity gave eroticism its savour of sin and legend when it endowed the human female with a soul; if society restores her sovereign individuality to woman, it will not thereby destroy the power of love's embrace to move the heart.

It is nonsense to assert that revelry, vice, ecstasy, passion, would become impossible if man and woman were equal in concrete matters; the contradictions that put the flesh in opposition to the spirit, the instant to time, the swoon of immanence to the challenge of transcendence, the absolute of pleasure to the nothingness of forgetting, will never be resolved; in sexuality will always be materialised the tension, the anguish, the joy, the frustration, and the triumph of existence. To emancipate woman is to refuse to confine her to the relations she bears to man, not to deny them to her; let her have her independent existence and she will continue none the less to exist for him also: mutually recognising each other as subject, each will yet remain for the other an other. The reciprocity of their relations will not do away with the miracles – desire, possession, love, dream, adventure – worked by the division of human beings into two separate categories; and the words that move us – giving, conquering, uniting – will not lose their meaning.

On the contrary, when we abolish the slavery of half of humanity, together with the whole system of hypocrisy that it implies, then the 'division' of humanity will reveal its genuine significance and the human couple will find its true form. 'The direct, natural, necessary relation of human creatures is *the relation of man to woman*,' Marx has said. 'The nature of this relation determines to what point man himself is to be considered as a *generic being*, as mankind; the relation of man to woman is the most natural relation of human being to human being. By it is shown, therefore, to what point the natural behaviour of man has become human or to what point the human being has become his *natural* being, to what point his human nature has become his *nature*.'

The case could not be better stated. It is for man to establish the reign of liberty in the midst of the world of the given. To gain the supreme victory, it is necessary, for one thing, that by and through their natural differentiation men and women unequivocally affirm their brotherhood.

The End.

On the publication of *The Second Sex*

The first volume of *The Second Sex* was published in June; in May, *Les Temps Modernes* had printed the chapter on 'Woman's Sexual Initiation' and followed it up in the June and July issues with the chapters on 'The Lesbian' and 'Maternity'. In November, Gallirnard published the second volume.

I have described how this book was first conceived, almost by chance. Wanting to talk about myself, I became aware that to do so I should first have to describe the condition of woman in *general;* first I considered the myths that men have forged about her through all their cosmologies, religions, superstitions, ideologies and literature. I tried to establish some order in the picture which at first appeared to me completely *incoherent*; in every case, man put himself forward as the Subject and considered the woman as an object, as the Other. This assumption could of course be explained by historical circumstances, and Sartre told me I should also give some indication of the physiological groundwork. That was at Ramatuelle; we talked about it for a long time and I hesitated; I hadn't expected to become involved in writing such a vast work. But it was true that my study of the myths would be left hanging in mid-air if people didn't know the reality those myths were intended to mask. I therefore plunged into works of physiology and history. I didn't merely compile; *even* scientists, of both sexes, are imbued with prejudices in favour of man, so I had to try to dig for the exact truth beneath the surface of their interpretations. From my journey into history I returned with a few ideas that I had never seen expressed anywhere: I linked the history of woman to that of inheritance, because it seemed to me to be a by-product of the economic evolution of the masculine world.

I began to look at women with new eyes and found surprise after surprise lying in wait for me. It is both strange and stimulating to discover suddenly, after forty, an aspect of the world that has been staring you in the face all the time which somehow you have never noticed. One of the misunderstandings created by my book is that people thought I was denying there was any difference between men and women. On the contrary, writing this book made me even more aware of those things that separate them; what I contended was that these dissimilarities are of a cultural and not of a natural order. I undertook to recount systematically, from childhood to old age, how they were created; I examined the possibilities this world offers women, those it denies them, their limits, their good and bad luck, their evasions and their achievements. That was what I put into the second volume: *L'Expérience vécue.*

I spent only two years on this, work.[1] already knew some sociology and psychology. Thanks to my university training, I had the habit of efficient working methods; I knew how to sort books out and strip the meat off them quickly, how to reject those that were merely rehashes of others or pure fantasies; I made a pretty exhaustive inventory of everything that had appeared on the subject in both English and French; it was one that had given rise to an enormous literature but, as is usually the case, only a small number of these studies were important. When it came to the second volume, I also profited from the continual interest that Sartre and I had had for so many years in all sorts of people; my memory provided me with an abundance of material.

The first volume was well received: twenty-two thousand copies were sold in the first week. The second one also sold well, but it shocked people. I was completely taken aback by the fuss it provoked when the extracts from the book appeared in *Les Temps Modernes*. I had completely failed to take into account that 'French bitchiness' Julien Gracq mentioned in an article in which – although he compared me to Poincaré making speeches in cemeteries – he congratulated me on my 'courage'. The word astonished me the first time it was used. 'How courageous you are!' Claudine Chonez told me with an admiration full of pity. 'Courageous?' 'You're going to lose a lot of friends!' Well, I thought to myself, if I lose them they're not friends. In any case, I had written this book just the way I wanted to write it, but there had been no thought of heroism in my mind at any time. The men whom I knew well – Sartre, Bost, Merleau-Ponty, Leiris, Giacometti and the staff of *Les Temps Modernes* – were real democrats on this point as well as on any other; if I had been writing it for them I would have been in danger of breaking down an open door. In any case I was accused of doing just that; also of inventing, parodying, digressing and ranting. I was accused of so many things: everything! First of all, indecency. The June, July and August issues of *Les Temps Modernes* sold like hot cakes; but they were read, as it were, with averted eyes. One might almost have believed that Freud and psychoanalysis had never existed. What a festival of obscenity on the pretext of flogging me for mine! That good old *esprit gaulois* flowed in torrents. I received some signed and some anonymous epigrams, epistles, satires, admonitions, and exhortations addressed to me by, for example, 'some very active members of the First Sex.' Unsatisfied, frigid, priapic, nymphomaniac, lesbian, a hundred times aborted, I was everything, even an unmarried mother. People offered to cure me of my frigidity or to temper my labial appetites; I was promised revelations, in the coarsest terms but in the name of the true, the good and the beautiful, in the name of health and even of poetry, all unworthily trampled underfoot by me. Certainly it is monotonous writing inscriptions on lavatory walls; I could understand that many sexual maniacs might prefer to send their lucubrations to me for a change. But I was a bit surprised at Mauriac! He wrote to one of the contributors to *Les Temps Modernes:* 'Your employer's vagina has no secrets from me,' which shows that in private life he wasn't afraid of words. When he saw them printed, it upset him so much that he began a series in *Le Figaro littéraire* urging the youth of France to condemn pornography in general and my articles in particular. Its success was slight. Although the replies of Pouillon and Cau, who had flown to my rescue, were suppressed – and probably those of many others as well – I had my defenders: among others, Domenach; the Christians were only gently indignant, and on the whole the youth of the nation did not seem excessively outraged by my verbal excesses. Mauriac lamented the fact bitterly. Exactly at the right moment to close his series, an angelic young lady sent him a letter so perfectly calculated to grant his every wish that a lot of us got a great deal of amusement out of what was obviously a godsend for Mauriac! Nevertheless, in restaurants and cafés – which I frequented much more than usual because of Algren – people often snickered as they glanced towards me or even openly pointed. Once, during an entire dinner at Nos Provinces on the Boulevard Montparnasse, a table of people nearby stared at me and giggled; I didn't like dragging Algren into a scene, but as I left I gave them a piece of my mind.

The violence and level of these reactions left me perplexed. Among the Latin peoples, Catholicism has encouraged masculine tyranny and even inclined it towards sadism; Italian men have a tendency to combine it with coarseness, and the Spaniards with arrogance, but this sort of meanness was particularly French. Why? Primarily because in France a man feels himself economically threatened by feminine competition; to maintain, or to assert the maintenance of a superiority no longer guaranteed by the customs of the country, the simplest method is to vilify women. A tradition of licentious talk provides a whole arsenal calculated to reduce women to their function as sexual objects: sayings, images, anecdotes and the vocabulary itself. Also, in the erotic field, the ancestral myth of French supremacy is being threatened; the ideal lover is now generally attributed to the Italian rather than the Frenchman; finally, the critical attitude of liberated women wounds or tires their partners; it makes them resentful. This meanness is simply the old French licentiousness taken over by vulnerable and spiteful men.[2]

In November, the swords were unsheathed once more. The critics went wild; there was no disagreement: women had always been the equal of men, they were forever doomed to be their inferiors, everything I said was common knowledge, there wasn't a word of truth in the whole book. In *Liberté de l'esprit,* Boideffre and Nimier outdid each other in contempt. I was a poor neurotic girl, repressed, frustrated, and cheated by life, a virago, a woman who'd never been made love to properly, envious, embittered and bursting with inferiority complexes with regard to men, while with regard to women I was eaten to the bone by resentment.[3] Jean Guitton, with great Christian compassion, wrote that *The Second Sex* had affected him painfully because one could so clearly see running through it the thread of 'my sad life'. Armand Hoog outdid himself: 'Humiliated by being a woman, agonizingly conscious of being imprisoned in her condition by the eyes of men, she rejects both their eyes and her condition.'

This theme of my humiliation was taken up by a considerable number of critics who were so naively imbued with their own masculine superiority that they could not even imagine that my condition had never been a burden to me. The man whom I placed above all others did not consider me inferior to men. I had many male friends whose eyes, far from imprisoning me within set limits, recognized me as a human being in my own right. Such good fortune had protected me against all resentment and all bitterness; my readers will know too that I was never infected by such feelings during my childhood or my adolescence.[4] Subtler readers concluded that I was a misogynist and that, while pretending to take up the cudgels for women, I was damning them; this is untrue. I do not praise them to the skies and I have anatomized all those defects engendered by their condition, but I also showed their good qualities and their merits. I have given too many women too much affection and esteem to betray them now by considering myself as an 'honorary male'; – nor have I ever been wounded by their stares. In fact I was never treated as a target for sarcasm until after *The Second Sex*; before that, people were either indifferent or kind to me. Afterwards, I was often attacked as a woman because my attackers thought it must be my Achilles' heel; but I knew perfectly well that this persistent petulance was really aimed at my moral and social convictions. No; far from suffering from my femininity, I have, on the contrary, from the age of twenty on, accumulated the advantages of both sexes; after *L'Invitée,* those around me treated me both as a writer, their peer in the masculine world, and as a woman; this was particularly noticeable in America: at the parties I went to, the wives all got together and talked to each other while I talked to the men, who nevertheless behaved towards me with greater courtesy than they did towards the members of their own sex. I was encouraged to write *The Second Sex* precisely because of this privileged position. It allowed me to express myself in all serenity. And, contrary to what they suggest, it was precisely this placidity which exasperated so many of my masculine readers. A wild cry of rage, the revolt of a wounded soul – that they could have accepted with a moved and pitying condescension; since they could not pardon me my objectivity, they feigned a disbelief in it. For example I will take a phrase of Claude Mauriac's which perfectly illustrates the arrogance of the First Sex. 'What has she got against me?' he wanted to know. Nothing; I had nothing against anything, except the words I was quoting. It is strange that so many intellectuals should refuse to believe in intellectual passions.[5]

I stirred up some storms even among my friends. One of them, a progressive academic, stopped reading my book and threw it across the room. Camus, in a few morose sentences, accused me of making the French male look ridiculous. A Mediterranean man, cultivating Spanish pride, he would allow woman equality only if she kept to her own, and different, realm; also, he was of course, as George Orwell would have said, the more equal of the two. He had blithely admitted to us once that he disliked the idea of being sized up and judged by a woman: she was the object, *he* was the eye and the consciousness. He laughed about it, but it is true that he did not accept reciprocity. Finally, with sudden warmth, he said: 'There's one argument that you should have emphasized: man himself suffers from not being able to find a real companion in woman; he does aspire to equality.' He too wanted a cry from the heart rather than solid reasoning; and what's more, a cry on behalf of men. Most men took as a personal insult the information I retailed about frigidity in women; they wanted to imagine that they could dispense pleasure whenever and to whomever they pleased; to doubt such powers on their part was to castrate them.

The Right could only detest my book, which Rome naturally put on the blacklist. I had hoped it would be well received by the extreme Left. Our relations with the Communists couldn't have been worse; all the same, my thesis owed so much to Marxism and showed it in such a favourable light that I did at least expect some impartiality from them! Marie-Louise Barron, in *Les Lettres françaises,* confined herself to remarking that *The Second Sex* would at least give the factory girls at Billancourt a good giggle; which implies a very low estimate of the factory girls at Billancourt, replied Colette Audry in a 'review of the critics' she did for *Combat Action* devoted an anonymous and unintelligible article to me, delightfully decorated with the photograph of a woman held fast in the passionate embraces of an ape.

The non-Stalinist Marxists were scarcely more comforting. I gave a lecture at the École Émancipée and was told that once the Revolution had been achieved, the problem of woman would no longer exist. Fine, I said; but meanwhile? The present apparently held no interest for them.

My adversaries created and maintained numerous misunderstandings on the subject of my book. Above all I was attacked for the chapter on maternity. Many men declared I had no right to discuss women because I hadn't given birth; and they?[6] They nevertheless produced some very distinct opinions of their own in opposition to mine. It was said that I refused to grant any value to the maternal instinct and to love. This was not so. I simply asked that women should experience them truthfully and freely, whereas they often use them as excuses and take refuge in them, only to find themselves imprisoned in that refuge when those emotions have dried up in their hearts. I was accused of preaching sexual promiscuity; but at no point did I ever advise anyone to sleep with just anyone at just any time; my opinion on this subject is that all choices, agreements and refusals should be made independently of institutions, conventions and motives of self-aggrandizement; if the reasons for it are not of the same order as the act itself, then the only result can be lies, distortions and mutilations.

I devoted a chapter to the problem of abortion; Sartre had already written about it in *The Age of Reason,* and I myself in *The Blood of Others;* people were always rushing into the office of *Les Temps Modernes* asking Mme Sorbets, the secretary, for addresses. She got so irritated that one day she designed a poster: WE DO IT ON THE PREMISES, OURSELVES. One morning, when I was still asleep, a young man knocked on my door. 'My wife is pregnant,' he said distractedly. 'Give me an address ...' 'But I don't know any,' I told him. He swore at me and left. 'No one ever helps anyone!' I didn't know any addresses; and I should scarcely have been inclined to have any confidence in a stranger endowed with so little self-control. Women and couples are forced by society into secrecy; if I can help them I have no hesitation in doing so. But I did not find it very pleasant to discover that I was apparently thought of as a professional procuress.

There were people who defended *The Second Sex:* Francis Jeanson, Nadeau, Mounier. It provoked public controversy and lectures, it brought me a considerable amount of correspondence. Misread and misunderstood, it troubled people's minds. When all is said and done, it is possibly the book that has brought me the greatest satisfaction of all those I have written. If I am asked what I think of it today, I have no hesitation in replying: I'm all for it.

Oh! I admit that one can criticize the style and the composition. I could easily go back and cut it down to a much more elegant work. But at the time I was discovering my ideas as I was explaining them, and that was the best I could do. As for the content, I should take a more materialist position today in the first volume. I should base the notion of woman as *other* and the Manichaean argument it entails not on an idealistic and *a priori* struggle of consciences, but on the facts of supply and demand; that is how I treated the same problem in *The Long March* when I was writing about the subjugation of women in ancient China. This modification would not necessitate any changes in the subsequent developments of my argument. On the whole, I still agree with what I said. I never cherished any illusion of changing woman's condition; it depends on the future of labour in the world; it will change significantly only at the price of a revolution in production. That is why I avoided falling into the trap of 'feminism'. Nor did I offer remedies for each particular problem I described. But at least I helped the women of my time and generation to become aware of themselves and their situation.

Many of them, of course, disapproved of my book; I disturbed them or opposed them or exasperated them or frightened them. But there were others to whom I did some service, as I know from numberless testimonies to the fact, especially from the letters that I am still receiving and answering after twelve years. These women have found help in my work in their fight against images of themselves which revolted them, against myths by which they felt themselves crushed; they came to realize that their difficulties reflected not a disgrace peculiar to them, but a general condition. This discovery helped them to avoid the mistake of self-contempt, and many of them found in the book the strength to fight against that condition. Self-knowledge is no guarantee of happiness, but it is on the side of happiness and can supply the courage to fight for it. Psychiatrists have told me that they give *The Second Sex* to their women patients to read, and not merely to intellectual women but to lower-middle-class women, to office workers and women working in factories. 'Your book was a great help to me. Your book saved me,' are the words I have read in letters from women of all ages and all walks of life.

If my book has helped women, it is because it expressed them, and they in their turn gave it its truth. Thanks to them, it is no longer a matter for scandal and concern. During these last ten years the myths that men created have crumbled, and many women writers have gone beyond me and have been far more daring than I. Too many of them for my taste take sexuality as their only theme; but at least when they write about it they now present themselves as the eye-that-looks, as subject, consciousness, freedom.

I should have been surprised and even irritated if, when I was thirty, someone had told me that I would be concerning myself with feminine problems, and that my most serious public would be made up of women. I don't regret that it has been so. Divided, lacerated, in a world made to put them at a disadvantage, for women there are far more victories to be won, more prizes to be gained, more defeats to he suffered than there are for men. I have an interest in them; and I prefer having taken a limited but real hold upon the world through them to drifting in the universal.

Footnotes

1. It was begun in October it 946 and finished in June 1949; but I spent four months of 1947 in America, and *America Day by Day* kept me busy for six months.

2. There exists a hatred of women among American men. But even the most venomous writings, such as Philip Wylie's *A Generation of Vipers,* do not descend to the level of obscenity; their sights are not on degrading women sexually.

3. When Christiane Rochefort's *Warrior's Rest* appeared ten years later, there was less scandal, but there were still plenty of male critics ready to chant the old refrain: 'She's an ugly and frustrated woman!'

4. I by no means despise resentment and bitterness, or any other of those negative emotions; they are often justified by circumstances and one might consider that I have missed something in not having experienced them. If I reject their attribution to me here it is because I would like *The Second Sex* to be understood in the spirit in which I wrote it.

5. A novelist pamphleteer of the Right, having been sharply attacked by Bost in *Les Temps Modernes*, exclaimed, very hurt: 'But why so much hate? He doesn't even know me!'

6. They went out and questioned mothers; but so did I.

The Ethics of Ambiguity

I. Ambiguity and Freedom

"Life in itself is neither good nor evil. It is the place of good and evil, according to what you make it." MONTAIGNE.

"THE continuous work of our life," says Montaigne, "is to build death." He quotes the Latin poets: *Prima, quae vitam dedit, hora corpsit.* And again: *Nascentes morimur.* Man knows and thinks this tragic ambivalence which the animal and the plant merely undergo. A new paradox is thereby introduced into his destiny. "Rational animal," "thinking reed," he escapes from his natural condition without, however, freeing himself from it. He is still a part of this world of which he is a consciousness. He asserts himself as a pure internality against which no external power can take hold, and he also experiences himself as a thing crushed by the dark weight of other things. At every moment he can grasp the non-temporal truth of his existence. But between the past which no longer is and the future which is not yet, this moment when he exists is nothing. This privilege, which he alone possesses, of being a sovereign and unique subject amidst a universe of objects, is what he shares with all his fellow-men. In turn an object for others, he is nothing more than an individual in the collectivity on which he depends.

As long as there have been men and they have lived, they have all felt this tragic ambiguity of their condition, but as long as there have been philosophers and they have thought, most of them have tried to mask it. They have striven to reduce mind to matter, or to reabsorb matter into mind, or to merge them within a single substance.

Those who have accepted the dualism have established a hierarchy between body and soul which permits of considering as negligible the part of the self which cannot be saved. They have denied death, either by integrating it with life or by promising to man immortality. Or, again they have denied life, considering it as a veil of illusion beneath which is hidden the truth of Nirvana.

And the ethics which they have proposed to their disciples has always pursued the same goal. It has been a matter of eliminating the ambiguity by making oneself pure inwardness or pure externality, by escaping from the sensible world or by being engulfed in it, by yielding to eternity or enclosing oneself in the pure moment. Hegel, with more ingenuity, tried to reject none of the aspects of man's condition and to reconcile them all. According to his system, the moment is preserved in the development of time; Nature asserts itself in the face of Spirit which denies it while assuming it; the individual is again found in the collectivity within which he is lost; and each man's death is fulfilled by being canceled out into the Life of Mankind. One can thus repose in a marvelous optimism where even the bloody wars simply express the fertile restlessness of the Spirit.

At the present time there still exist many doctrines which choose to leave in the shadow certain troubling aspects of a too complex situation. But their attempt to lie to us is in vain. Cowardice doesn't pay. Those reasonable metaphysics, those consoling ethics with which they would like to entice us only accentuate the disorder from which we suffer. Men of today seem to feel more acutely than ever the paradox of their condition. They know themselves to be the supreme end to which all action should be subordinated, but the exigencies of action force them to treat one another as instruments or obstacles, as means. The more widespread their mastery of the world, the more they find themselves crushed by uncontrollable forces. Though they are masters of the atomic bomb, yet it is created only to destroy them. Each one has the incomparable taste in his mouth of his own life, and yet each feels himself more insignificant than an insect within the immense collectivity whose limits are one with the earth's. Perhaps in no other age have they manifested their grandeur more brilliantly, and in no other age has this grandeur been so horribly flouted. In spite of so many stubborn lies, at every moment, at every opportunity, the truth comes to light, the truth of life and death, of my solitude and my bond with the world, of my freedom and my servitude, of the insignificance and the sovereign importance of each man and all men. There was Stalingrad and there was Buchenwald, and neither of the two wipes out the other. Since we do not succeed in fleeing it, let us therefore try to look the truth in the face. Let us try to assume our fundamental ambiguity. It is in the knowledge of the genuine conditions of our life that we must draw our strength to live and our reason for acting.

From the very beginning, existentialism defined itself as a philosophy of ambiguity. It was by affirming the irreducible character of ambiguity that Kierkegaard opposed himself to Hegel, and it is by ambiguity that, in our own generation, Sartre, in *Being and Nothingness,* fundamentally defined man, that being whose being is not to be, that subjectivity which realizes itself only as a presence in the world, that engaged freedom, that surging of the for-oneself which is immediately given for others. But it is also claimed that existentialism is a philosophy of the absurd and of despair. It encloses man in a sterile anguish, in an empty subjectivity. It is incapable of furnishing him with any principle for making choices. Let him do as he pleases. In any case, the game is lost. Does not Sartre declare, in effect, that man is a "useless passion," that he tries in vain to realize the synthesis of the for-oneself and the in-oneself, to make himself God? It is true. But it is also true that the most optimistic ethics have all begun by emphasizing the element of failure involved in the condition of man; without failure, no ethics; for a being who, from the very start, would be an exact co-incidence with himself, in a perfect plenitude, the notion of having-to-be would have no meaning. One does not offer an ethics to a God. It is impossible to propose any to man if one defines him as nature, as something given. The so-called psychological or empirical ethics manage to establish themselves only by introducing surreptitiously some flaw within the manthing which they have first defined. Hegel tells us in the last part of *The Phenomenology of Mind* that moral consciousness can exist only to the extent that there is disagreement between nature and morality. It would disappear if the ethical law became the natural law. To such an extent that by a paradoxical "displacement," if moral action is the absolute goal, the absolute goal is also that moral action may not be present. This means that there can be a having-to-be only for a being who, according to the existentialist definition, questions himself in his being, a being who is at a distance from himself and who has to be his being.

Well and good. But it is still necessary for the failure to be surmounted, and existentialist ontology does not allow this hope. Man's passion is useless; he has no means for becoming the being that he is not. That too is true. And it is also true that in *Being and Nothingness* Sartre has insisted above all on the abortive aspect of the human adventure. It is only in the last pages that he opens up the perspective for an ethics. However, if we reflect upon his descriptions of existence, we perceive that they are far from condemning man without recourse.

The failure described in *Being and Nothingness* is definitive, but it is also ambiguous. Man, Sartre tells us, is "a being who *makes himself* a lack of being *in order that there might be* being." That means, first of all, that his passion is not inflicted upon him from without. He chooses it. It is his very being and, as such, does not imply the idea of unhappiness. If this choice is considered as useless, it is because there exists no absolute value before the passion of man, outside of it, in relation to which one might distinguish the useless from the useful. The word "useful" has not yet received a meaning on the level of description where *Being and Nothingness* is situated. It can be defined only in the human world established by man's projects and the ends he sets up. In the original helplessness from which man surges up, nothing is useful, nothing is useless. It must therefore be understood that the passion to which man has acquiesced finds no external justification. No outside appeal, no objective necessity permits of its being called useful. It has no reason to will itself. But this does not mean that it can not justify itself, that it can not *give itself* reasons for being that it does not *have*. And indeed Sartre tells us that man makes himself this lack of being *in order that* there might be being. The term *in order that* clearly indicates an intentionality. It is not in vain that man nullifies being. Thanks to him, being is disclosed and he desires this disclosure. There is an original type of attachment to being which is not the relationship "wanting to be" but rather "wanting to disclose being." Now, here there is not failure, but rather success. This end, which man proposes to himself by making himself lack of being, is, in effect, realized by him. By uprooting himself from the world, man makes himself present to the world and makes the world present to him. I should like to be the landscape which I am contemplating, I should like this sky, this quiet water to think themselves within me, that it might be I whom they express in flesh and bone, and I remain at a distance. But it is also by this distance that the sky and the water exist before me. My contemplation is an excruciation only because it is also a joy. I can not appropriate the snow field where I slide. It remains foreign, forbidden, but I take delight in this very effort toward an impossible possession. I experience it as a triumph, not as a defeat. This means that man, in his vain attempt to *be* God, makes himself exist as man, and if he is satisfied with this existence, he coincides exactly with himself. It is not granted him to exist without tending toward this being which he will never be. But it is possible for him to want this tension even with the failure which it involves. His being is lack of being, but this lack has a way of being which is precisely existence. In Hegelian terms it might be said that we have here a negation of the negation by which the positive is re-established. Man makes himself a lack, but he can deny the lack as lack and affirm himself as a positive existence. He then assumes the failure. And the condemned action, insofar as it is an effort to be, finds its validity insofar as it is a manifestation of existence. However, rather than being a Hegelian act of surpassing, it is a matter of a conversion. For in Hegel the surpassed terms are preserved only as abstract moments, whereas we consider that existence still remains a negativity in the positive affirmation of itself. And it does not appear, in its turn, as the term of a further synthesis. The failure is not surpassed, but assumed. Existence asserts itself as an absolute which must seek its justification within itself and not suppress itself, even though it may be lost by preserving itself. To attain his truth, man must not attempt to dispel the ambiguity of his being but, on the contrary, accept the task of realizing it. He rejoins himself only to the extent that he agrees to remain at a distance from himself. This conversion is sharply distinguished from the Stoic conversion in that it does not claim to oppose to the sensible universe a formal freedom which is without content. To exist genuinely is not to deny this spontaneous movement of my transcendence, but only to refuse to lose myself in it. Existentialist conversion should rather be compared to Husserlian reduction: let man put his will to be "in parentheses" and he will thereby be brought to the consciousness of his true condition. And just as phenomenological reduction prevents the errors of dogmatism by suspending all affirmation concerning the mode of reality of the external world, whose flesh and bone presence the reduction does not, however, contest, so existentialist conversion does not suppress my instincts, desires, plans, and passions. It merely prevents any possibility of failure by refusing to set up as absolutes the ends toward which my transcendence thrusts itself, and by considering them in their connection with the freedom which projects them.

The first implication of such an attitude is that the genuine man will not agree to recognize any foreign absolute. When a man projects into an ideal heaven that impossible synthesis of the for-itself and the in-itself that is called God, it is because he wishes the regard of this existing Being to change his existence into being; but if he agrees not to be in order to exist genuinely, he will abandon the dream of an inhuman objectivity. He will understand that it is not a matter of being right in the eyes of a God, but of being right in his own eyes. Renouncing the thought of seeking the guarantee for his existence outside of himself, he will also refuse to believe in unconditioned values which would set themselves up athwart his freedom like things. Value is this lacking-being of which freedom *makes itself* a lack; and it is because the latter makes itself a lack that value appears. It is desire which creates the desirable, and the project which sets up the end. It is human existence which makes values spring up in the world on the basis of which it will be able to judge the enterprise in which it will be engaged. But first it locates itself beyond any pessimism, as beyond any optimism, for the fact of its original springing forth is a pure contingency. Before existence there is no more reason to exist than not to exist. The lack of existence can not be evaluated since it is the fact on the basis of which all evaluation is defined. It can not be compared to anything for there is nothing outside of it to serve as a term of comparison. This rejection of any extrinsic justification also confirms the rejection of an original pessimism which we posited at the beginning. Since it is unjustifiable from without, to declare from without that it is unjustifiable is not to condemn it. And the truth is that outside of existence there is nobody. Man exists. For him it is not a question of wondering whether his presence in the world is useful, whether life is worth the trouble of being lived. These questions make no sense. It is a matter of knowing whether he wants to live and under what conditions.

But if man is free to define for himself the conditions of a life which is valid in his own eyes, can he not choose whatever he likes and act however he likes? Dostoevsky asserted, "If God does not exist, everything is permitted." Today's believers use this formula for their own advantage. To re-establish man at the heart of his destiny is, they claim, to repudiate all ethics. However, far from God's absence authorizing all license, the contrary is the case, because man is abandoned on the earth, because his acts are definitive, absolute engagements. He bears the responsibility for a world which is not the work of a strange power, but of himself, where his defeats are inscribed, and his victories as well. A God can pardon, efface, and compensate. But if God does not exist, man's faults are inexpiable. If it is claimed that, whatever the case may be, this earthly stake has no importance, this is precisely because one invokes that inhuman objectivity which we declined at the start. One can not start by saying that our earthly destiny *has* or *has not* importance, for it depends upon us to give it importance. It is up to man to make it important to be a man, and he alone can feel his success or failure. And if it is again said that nothing forces him to try to justify his being in this way, then one is playing upon the notion of freedom in a dishonest way. The believer is also free to sin. The divine law is imposed upon him only from the moment he decides to save his soul. In the Christian religion, though one speaks very little about them today, there are also the damned. Thus, on the earthly plane, a life which does not seek to ground itself will be a pure contingency. But it is permitted to wish to give itself a meaning and a truth, and it then meets rigorous demands within its own heart.

However, even among the proponents of secular ethics, there are many who charge existentialism with offering no objective content to the moral act. It is said that this philosophy is subjective, even solipsistic. If he is once enclosed within himself, how can man get out? But there too we have a great deal of dishonesty. It is rather well known that the fact of being a subject is a universal fact and that the Cartesian *cogito* expresses both the most individual experience and the most objective truth. By affirming that the source of all values resides in the freedom of man, existentialism merely carries on the tradition of Kant, Fichte, and Hegel, who, in the words of Hegel himself, "have taken for their point of departure the principle according to which the essence of right and duty and the essence of the thinking and willing subject are absolutely identical." The idea that defines all humanism is that the world is not a given world, foreign to man, one to which he has to force himself to yield without. It is the world willed by man, insofar as his will expresses his genuine reality.

Some will answer, "All well and good. But Kant escapes solipsism because for him genuine reality is the human person insofar as it transcends its empirical embodiment and chooses to be universal." And doubtless Hegel asserted that the "right of individuals to their particularity is equally contained in ethical substantiality, since particularity is the extreme, phenomenal modality in which moral reality exists (*Philosophy of Right, ?* 154)." But for him particularity appears only as a moment of the totality in which it must surpass itself. Whereas for existentialism, it is not impersonal universal man who is the source of values, but the plurality of concrete – particular men projecting themselves toward their ends on the basis of situations whose particularity is as radical and as irreducible as subjectivity itself. How could men, originally separated, get together?

And, indeed, we are coming to the real situation of the problem. But to state it is not to demonstrate that it can not be resolved. On the contrary, we must here again invoke the notion of Hegelian "displacement." There is an ethics only if there is a problem to solve. And it can be said, by inverting the preceding line of argument, that the ethics which have given solutions by effacing the fact of the separation of men are not valid precisely because there is this separation. An ethics of ambiguity will be one which will refuse to deny *a priori* that separate existants can, at the same time, be bound to each other, that their individual freedoms can forge laws valid for all.

Before undertaking the quest for a solution, it is interesting to note that the notion of situation and the recognition of separation which it implies are not peculiar to existentialism. We also meet it in Marxism which, from one point of view, can be considered as an apotheosis of subjectivity. Like all radical humanism, Marxism rejects the idea of an inhuman objectivity and locates itself in the tradition of Kant and Hegel. Unlike the old kind of utopian socialism which confronted earthly order with the archetypes of justice, Order, and Good, Marx does not consider that certain human situations are, in themselves and absolutely, preferable to others. It is the needs of people, the revolt of a class, which define aims and goals. It is from within a rejected situation, in the light of this rejection, that a new state appears as desirable; only the will of men decides; and it is on the basis of a certain individual act of rooting itself in the historical and economic world that this will thrusts itself, toward the future and then chooses a perspective where such words as goal, progress, efficacy, success, failure, action, adversaries, instruments, and obstacles, have a meaning. Then certain acts can be regarded as good and others as bad.

In order for the universe of revolutionary values to arise, a subjective movement must create them in revolt and hope. And this movement appears so essential to Marxists that if an intellectual or a bourgeois also claims to want revolution, they distrust him. They think that it is only from the outside, by abstract recognition, that the bourgeois intellectual can adhere to these values which he himself has not set up. Regardless of what he does, his situation makes it impossible for the ends pursued by proletarians to be absolutely his ends too, since it is not the very impulse of his life which has begotten them.

However, in Marxism, if it is true that the goal and the meaning of action are defined by human wills, these wills do not appear as free. They are the reflection of objective conditions by which the situation of the class or the people under consideration is defined. In the present moment of the development of capitalism, the proletariat can not help wanting its elimination as a class. Subjectivity is re-absorbed into the objectivity of the given world. Revolt, need, hope, rejection, and desire are only the resultants of external forces. The psychology of behavior endeavors to explain this alchemy.

It is known that that is the essential point on which existentialist ontology is opposed to dialectical materialism. We think that the meaning of the situation does not impose itself on the consciousness of a passive subject, that it surges up only by the disclosure which a free subject effects in his project. It appears evident to us that in order to adhere to Marxism, to enroll in a party, and in one rather than another, to be actively attached to it, even a Marxist needs a decision whose source is only in himself. And this autonomy is not the privilege (or the defect) of the intellectual or- the bourgeois. The proletariat, taken as a whole, as a class, can become conscious of its situation in more than one way. It can want the revolution to be brought about by one party or another. It can let itself be lured on, as happened to the German proletariat, or can sleep in the dull comfort which capitalism grants it, as does the American proletariat. It may be said that in all these cases it is betraying; still, it must be free to betray. Or, if one pretends to distinguish the real proletariat from a treacherous proletariat, or a misguided or unconscious or mystified one, then it is no longer a flesh and blood proletariat that one is dealing with, but the idea of a proletariat, one of those ideas which Marx ridiculed.

Besides, in practice, Marxism does not always deny freedom. The very notion of action would lose all meaning if history were a mechanical unrolling in which man appears only as a passive conductor of outside forces. By acting, as also by preaching action, the Marxist revolutionary asserts himself as a veritable agent; he assumes himself to be free. And it is even curious to note that most Marxists of today - unlike Marx himself - feel no repugnance at the edifying dullness of moralizing speeches. They do not limit themselves to finding fault with their adversaries in the name of historical realism. When they tax them with cowardice, lying, selfishness, and venality, they very well mean to condemn them in the name of a moralism superior to history. Likewise, in the eulogies which they bestow upon each other they exalt the eternal virtues, courage, abnegation, lucidity, integrity. It may be said that all these words are used for propagandistic purposes, that it is only a matter of expedient language. But this is to admit that this language is heard, that it awakens an echo in the hearts of those to whom it is addressed. Now, neither scorn nor esteem would have any meaning if one regarded the acts of a man as a purely mechanical resultant. In order for men to become indignant or to admire, they must be conscious of their own freedom and the freedom of others. Thus, everything occurs within each man and in the collective tactics as if men were free. But then what revelation can a coherent humanism hope to oppose to the testimony which man brings to bear upon himself? So Marxists often find themselves having to confirm this belief in freedom, even if they have to reconcile it with determination as well as they can.

However, while this concession is wrested from them by the very practice of action, it is in the name of action that they attempt to condemn a philosophy of freedom. They declare authoritatively that the existence of freedom would make any concerted enterprise impossible. According to them, if the individual were not constrained by the external world to want this rather than that, there would be nothing to defend him against his whims. Here, in different language, we again meet the charge formulated by the respectful believer of supernatural imperatives. In the eyes of the Marxist, as of the Christian, it seems that to act freely is to give up justifying one's acts. This is a curious reversal of the Kantian "you must; therefore you can," Kant postulates freedom in the name of morality. The Marxist, on the contrary, declares, "You must; therefore, you can not." To him a man's action seems valid only if the man has not helped set it going by an internal movement. To admit the ontological possibility of a choice is already to betray the Cause. Does this mean that the revolutionary attitude in any way gives up being a moral attitude? It would be logical, since we observed with Hegel that it is only insofar as the choice is not realized at first that it can be set up as a moral choice. But here again Marxist thought hesitates. It sneers at idealistic ethics which do not bite into the world; but its scoffing signifies that there can be no ethics outside of action, not that action lowers itself to the level of a simple natural process. It is quite evident that the revolutionary enterprise has a human meaning. Lenin's remark[1], which says, in substance, "I call any action useful to the party moral action; I call it immoral if it is harmful to the party," cuts two ways. On the one hand, he refuses to accept outdated values, but he also sees in political operation a total manifestation of man as having-to-be at the same time as being. Lenin refuses to set up ethics abstractly because he means to realize it effectively. And yet a moral idea is present in the words, writings, and acts of Marxists. It is contradictory, then, to reject with horror the moment of choice which is precisely the moment when spirit passes into nature, the moment of the concrete fulfillment of man and morality.

As for us, whatever the case may be, we believe in freedom. Is it true that this belief must lead us to despair? Must we grant this curious paradox: that from the moment a man recognizes himself as free, he is prohibited from wishing for anything?

On the contrary, it appears to us that by turning toward this freedom we are going to discover a principle of action whose range will be universal. The characteristic feature of all ethics is to consider human life as a game that can be won or lost and to teach man the means of winning. Now, we have seen that the original scheme of man is ambiguous: he wants to be, and to the extent that he coincides with this wish, he fails. All the plans in which this will to be is actualized are condemned; and the ends circumscribed by these plans remain mirages. Human transcendence is vainly engulfed in those miscarried attempts. But man also wills himself to be a disclosure of being, and if he coincides with this wish, he wins, for the fact is that the world becomes present by his presence in it. But the disclosure implies a perpetual tension to keep being at a certain distance, to tear one self from the world, and to assert oneself as a freedom. To wish for the disclosure of the world and to assert oneself as freedom are one and the same movement. Freedom is the source from which all significations and all values spring. It is the original condition of all justification of existence. The man who seeks to justify his life must want freedom itself absolutely and above everything else. At the same time that it requires the realization of concrete ends, of particular projects, it requires itself universally. It is not a ready-made value which offers itself from the outside to my abstract adherence, but it appears (not on the plane of facility, but on the moral plane) as a cause of itself. It is necessarily summoned up by the values which it sets up and through which it sets itself up. It can not establish a denial of itself, for in denying itself, it would deny the possibility of any foundation. To will oneself moral and to will oneself free are one and the same decision.

It seems that the Hegelian notion of "displacement" which we relied on a little while ago is now turning against us. There is ethics only if ethical action is not present. Now, Sartre declares that every man is free, that there is no way of his not being free. When he wants to escape his destiny, he is still freely fleeing it. Does not this presence of a so to speak natural freedom contradict the notion of ethical freedom? What meaning can there be in the words *to will oneself free,* since at the beginning we *are* free? It is contradictory to set freedom up as something conquered if at first it is something given.

This objection would mean something only if freedom were a thing or a quality naturally attached to a thing. Then, in effect, one would either have it or not have it. But the fact is that it merges with the very movement of this ambiguous reality which is called existence and which is only by making itself be; to such an extent that it is precisely only by having to be conquered that it gives itself. To will oneself free is to effect the transition from nature to morality by establishing a genuine freedom on the original upsurge of our existence.

Every man is originally free, in the sense that he spontaneously casts himself into the world. But if we consider this spontaneity in its facticity, it appears to us only as a pure contingency, an upsurging as stupid as the clinamen of the Epicurean atom which turned up at any moment whatsoever from any direction whatsoever. And it was quite necessary for the atom to arrive somewhere. But its movement was not justified by this result which had not been chosen. It remained absurd. Thus, human spontaneity always projects itself toward something. The psychoanalyst discovers a meaning even in abortive acts and attacks of hysteria. But in order for this meaning to justify the transcendence which discloses it, it must itself be founded, which it will never be if I do not choose to found it myself. Now, I can evade this choice. We have said that it would be contradictory deliberately to will oneself not free. But one can choose not to will himself free. In laziness, heedlessness, capriciousness, cowardice, impatience, one contests the meaning of the project at the very moment that one defines it. The spontaneity of the subject is then merely a vain living palpitation, its movement toward the object is a flight, and itself is an absence. To convert the absence into presence, to convert my flight into will, I must assume my project positively. It is not a matter of retiring into the completely inner and, moreover, abstract movement of a given spontaneity, but of adhering to the concrete and particular movement by which this spontaneity defines itself by thrusting itself toward an end. It is through this end that it sets up that my spontaneity confirms itself by reflecting upon itself. Then, by a single movement, my will, establishing the content of the act, is legitimized by it. I realize my escape toward the other as a freedom when, assuming the presence of the object, I thereby assume myself before it as a presence. But this justification requires a constant tension. My project is never founded; it founds itself. To avoid the anguish of this permanent choice, one may attempt to flee into the object itself, to engulf one's own presence in it. In the servitude of the serious, the original spontaneity strives to deny itself. It strives in vain, and meanwhile it then fails to fulfill itself as moral freedom.

We have just described only the subjective and formal aspect of this freedom. But we also ought to ask ourselves whether one can will oneself free in any matter, whatsoever it may be. It must first be observed that this will is developed in the course of time. It is in time that the goal is pursued and that freedom confirms itself. And this assumes that it is realized as a unity in the unfolding of time. One escapes the absurdity of the clinamen only by escaping the absurdity of the pure moment. An existence would be unable to found itself if moment by moment it crumbled into nothingness. That is why no moral question presents itself to the child as long as he is still incapable of recognizing himself in the past or seeing himself in the future. It is only when the moments of his life begin to be organized into behaviour that he can decide and choose. The value of the chosen end is confined and, reciprocally, the genuineness of the choice is manifested concretely through patience, courage, and fidelity. If I leave behind an act which I have accomplished, it becomes a thing by falling into the past. It is no longer anything but a stupid and opaque fact. In order to prevent this metamorphosis, I must ceaselessly return to it and justify it in the unity of the project in which I am engaged. Setting up the movement of my transcendence requires that I never let it uselessly fall back upon itself, that I prolong it indefinitely. Thus I can not genuinely desire an end today without desiring it through my whole existence, insofar as it is the future of this present moment and insofar as it is the surpassed past of days to come. To will is to engage myself to persevere in my will. This does not mean that I ought not aim at any limited end. I may desire absolutely and forever a revelation of a moment. This means that the value of this provisional end will be confirmed indefinitely. But this living confirmation can not be merely contemplative and verbal. It is carried out in an act. The goal toward which I surpass myself must appear to me as a point of departure toward a new act of surpassing. Thus, a creative freedom develops happily without ever congealing into unjustified facticity. The creator leans upon anterior creations in order to create the possibility of new creations. His present project embraces the past and places confidence in the freedom to come, a confidence which is never disappointed. It discloses being at the end of a further disclosure. At each moment freedom is confirmed through all creation.

However, man does not create the world. He succeeds in disclosing it only through the resistance which the world opposes to him. The will is defined only by raising obstacles, and by the contingency of facticity certain obstacles let themselves be conquered, and others do not. This is what Descartes expressed when he said that the freedom of man is infinite, but his power is limited. How can the presence of these limits be reconciled with the idea of a freedom confirming itself as a unity and an indefinite movement?

In the face of an obstacle which it is impossible to overcome, stubbornness is stupid. If I persist in beating my fist against a stone wall, my freedom exhausts itself in this useless gesture without succeeding in giving itself a content. It debases itself in a vain contingency. Yet, there is hardly a sadder virtue than resignation. It transforms into phantoms and contingent reveries projects which had at the beginning been set up as will and freedom. A young man has hoped for a happy or useful or glorious life. If the man he has become looks upon these miscarried attempts of his adolescence with disillusioned indifference, there they are, forever frozen in the dead past. When an effort fails, one declares bitterly that he has lost time and wasted his powers. The failure condemns that whole part of ourselves which we had engaged in the effort. It was to escape this dilemma that the Stoics preached indifference. We could indeed assert our freedom against all constraint if we agreed to renounce the particularity of our projects. If a door refuses to open, let us accept not opening it and there we are free. But by doing that, one manages only to save an abstract notion of freedom. It is emptied of all content and all truth. The power of man ceases to be limited because it is annulled. It is the particularity of the project which determines the limitation of the power, but it is also what gives the project its content and permits it to be set up. There are people who are filled with such horror at the idea of a defeat that they keep themselves from ever doing anything. But no one would dream of considering this gloomy passivity as the triumph of freedom.

The truth is that in order for my freedom not to risk coming to grief against the obstacle which its very engagement has raised, in order that it might still pursue its movement in the face of the failure, it must, by giving itself a particular content, aim by means of it at an end which is nothing else but precisely the free movement of existence. Popular opinion is quite right in admiring a man who, having been ruined or having suffered an accident, knows how to gain the upper hand, that is, renew his engagement in the world, thereby strongly asserting the independence of freedom in relation to thing. Thus, when the sick Van Gogh calmly accepted the prospect of a future in which he would be unable to paint any more, there was no sterile resignation. For him painting was a personal way of life and of communication with others which in another form could be continued even in an asylum. The past will be integrated and freedom will be confirmed in a renunciation of this kind. It will be lived in both heartbreak and joy. In heartbreak, because the project is then robbed of its particularity - it sacrifices its flesh and blood. But in joy, since at the moment one releases his hold, he again finds his hands free and ready to stretch out toward a new future. But this act of passing beyond is conceivable only if what the content has in view is not to bar up the future, but, on the contrary, to plan new possibilities. This brings us back by another route to what we had already indicated. My freedom must not seek to trap being but to disclose it. The disclosure is the transition from being to existence. The goal which my freedom aims at is conquering existence across the always inadequate density of being.

However, such salvation is only possible if, despite obstacles and failures, a man preserves the disposal of his future, if the situation opens up more possibilities to him. In case his transcendence is cut off from his goal or there is no longer any hold on objects which might give it a valid content, his spontaneity is dissipated without founding anything. Then he may not justify his existence positively and he feels its contingency with wretched disgust. There is no more obnoxious way to punish a man than to force him to perform acts which make no sense to him, as when one empties and fills the same ditch indefinitely, when one makes soldiers who are being punished march up and down, or when one forces a schoolboy to copy lines. Revolts broke out in Italy in September 1946 because the unemployed were set to breaking pebbles which served no purpose whatever. As is well known, this was also the weakness which ruined the national workshops in 1848. This mystification of useless effort is more intolerable than fatigue. Life imprisonment is the most horrible of punishments because it preserves existence in its pure facticity but forbids it all legitimation. A freedom can not will itself without willing itself as an indefinite movement. It must absolutely reject the constraints which arrest its drive toward itself. This rejection takes on a positive aspect when the constraint is natural. One rejects the illness by curing it. But it again assumes the negative aspect of revolt when the oppressor is a human freedom. One can not deny being: the in-itself is, and negation has no hold over this being, this pure positivity; one does not escape this fullness: a destroyed house is a ruin; a broken chain is scrap iron: one attains only signification and, through it, the for-itself which is projected there; the for-itself carries nothingness in its heart and can be annihilated, whether in the very upsurge of its existence or through the world in which it exists. The prison is repudiated as such when the prisoner escapes. But revolt, insofar as it is pure negative movement, remains abstract. It is fulfilled as freedom only by returning to the positive, that is, by giving itself a content through action, escape, political struggle, revolution. Human transcendence then seeks, with the destruction of the given situation, the whole future which will flow from its victory. It resumes its indefinite rapport with itself. There are limited situations where this return to the positive is impossible, where the future is radically blocked off. Revolt can then be achieved only in the definitive rejection of the imposed situation, in suicide.

It can be seen that, on the one hand, freedom can always save itself, for it is realized as a disclosure of existence through its very failures, and it can again confirm itself by a death freely chosen. But, on the other hand, the situations which it discloses through its project toward itself do not appear as equivalents. It regards as privileged situations those which permit it to realize itself as indefinite movement; that is, it wishes to pass beyond everything which limits its power; and yet, this power is always limited. Thus, just as life is identified with the will-to-live, freedom always appears as a movement of liberation. It is only by prolonging itself through the freedom of others that it manages to surpass death itself and to realize itself as an indefinite unity. Later on we shall see what problems such a relationship raises. For the time being it is enough for us to have established the fact that the words "to will oneself free" have a positive and concrete meaning. If man wishes to save his existence, as only he himself can do, his original spontaneity must be raised to the height of moral freedom by taking itself as an end through the disclosure of a particular content.

But a new question is immediately raised. If man has one and only one way to save his existence, how can he choose not to choose it in all cases? How is a bad willing possible? We meet with this problem in all ethics, since it is precisely the possibility of a perverted willing which gives a meaning to the idea of virtue. We know the answer of Socrates, of Plato, of Spinoza: "No one is willfully bad." And if Good is a transcendent thing which is more or less foreign to man, one imagines that the mistake can be explained by error. But if one grants that the moral world is the world genuinely willed by man, all possibility of error is eliminated. Moreover, in Kantian ethics, which is at the origin of all ethics of autonomy, it is very difficult to account for an evil will. As the choice of his character which the subject makes is achieved in the intelligible world by a purely rational will, one can not understand how the latter expressly rejects the law which it gives to itself. But this is because Kantism defined man as a pure positivity, and it therefore recognized no other possibility in him than coincidence with himself. We, too, define morality by this adhesion to the self; and this is why we say that man can not positively decide between the negation and the assumption of his freedom, for as soon as he decides, he assumes it. He can not positively will not to be free for such a willing would be self-destructive. Only, unlike Kant, we do not see man as being essentially a positive will. On the contrary, he is first defined as a negativity. He is first at a distance from himself. He can coincide with himself only by agreeing never to rejoin himself. There is within him a perpetual playing with the negative, and he thereby escapes himself, he escapes his freedom. And it is precisely because an evil will is here possible that the words "to will oneself free" have a meaning. Therefore, not only do we assert that the existentialist doctrine permits the elaboration of an ethics, but it even appears to us as the only philosophy in which an ethics has its place. For, in a metaphysics of transcendence, in the classical sense of the term, evil is reduced to error; and in humanistic philosophies it is impossible to account for it, man being defined as complete in a complete world. Existentialism alone gives - like religions - a real role to evil, and it is this, perhaps, which make its judgments so gloomy. Men do not like to feel themselves in danger. Yet, it is because there are real dangers, real failures and real earthly damnation that words like victory, wisdom, or joy have meaning. Nothing is decided in advance, and it is because man has something to lose and because he can lose that he can also win.

Therefore, in the very condition of man there enters the possibility of not fulfilling this condition. In order to fulfill it he must assume himself as a being who "makes himself a lack of being so that there might be being." But the trick of dishonesty permits stopping at any moment whatsoever. One may hesitate to make oneself a lack of being, one may withdraw before existence, or one may falsely assert oneself as being, or assert oneself as nothingness. One may realize his freedom only as an abstract independence, or, on the contrary, reject with despair the distance which separates us from being. All errors are possible since man is a negativity, and they are motivated by the anguish he feels in the face of his freedom. Concretely, men slide incoherently from one attitude to another. We shall limit ourselves to describing in their abstract form those which we have just indicated.

II. Personal Freedom and Others

Man's unhappiness, says Descartes, is due to his having first been a child. And indeed the unfortunate choices which most men make can only be explained by the fact that they have taken place on the basis of childhood. The child's situation is characterized by his finding himself cast into a universe which he has not helped to establish, which has been fashioned without him, and which appears to him as an absolute to which he can only submit. In his eyes, human inventions, words, customs, and values are given facts, as inevitable as the sky and the trees. This means that the world in which he lives is a serious world, since the characteristic of the spirit of seriousness is to consider values as ready-made things. That does not mean that the child himself is serious. On the contrary, he is allowed to play, to expend his existence freely. In his child's circle he feels that he can passionately pursue and joyfully attain goals which he has set up for himself. But if he fulfills this experience in all tranquillity, it is precisely because the domain open to his subjectivity seems insignificant and puerile in his own eyes. He feels himself happily irresponsible. The real world is that of adults where he is allowed only to respect and obey. The naive victim of the mirage of the for-others, he believes in the being of his parents and teachers. He takes them for the divinities which they vainly try to be and whose appearance they like to borrow before his ingenuous eyes. Rewards, punishments, prizes, words of praise or blame instill in him the conviction that there exist a good and an evil which like a sun and a moon exist as ends in themselves. In his universe of definite and substantial things, beneath the sovereign eyes of grown-up persons, he thinks that he too has *BEING* in a definite and substantial way. He is a good little boy or a scamp; he enjoys being it. If something deep inside him belies his conviction, he conceals this imperfection. He consoles himself for an inconsistency which he attributes to his young age by pinning his hopes on the future. Later on he too will become a big imposing statue. While waiting, he plays at being, at being a saint, a hero, a guttersnipe. He feels himself like those models whose images are sketched out in his books in broad, unequivocal strokes: explorer, brigand, sister of charity. This game of being serious can take on such an importance in the child's life that he himself actually becomes serious. We know such children who are caricatures of adults. Even when the joy of existing is strongest, when the child abandons himself to it, he feels himself protected against the risk of existence by the ceiling which human generations have built over his head. And it is by virtue of this that the child's condition (although it can be unhappy in other respects) is metaphysically privileged. Normally the child escapes the anguish of freedom. He can, if he likes, be recalcitrant, lazy; his whims and his faults concern only him. They do not weigh upon the earth. They can not make a dent in the serene order of a world which existed before him, without him, where he is in a state of security by virtue of his very insignificance. He can do with impunity whatever he likes. He knows that nothing can ever happen through him; everything is already given; his acts engage nothing, not even himself.

There are beings whose life slips by in an infantile world because, having been kept in a state of servitude and ignorance, they have no means of breaking the ceiling which is stretched over their heads. Like the child, they can exercise their freedom, but only within this universe which has been set up before them, without them. This is the case, for example, of slaves who have not raised themselves to the consciousness of their slavery. The southern planters were not altogether in the wrong in considering the negroes who docilely submitted to their paternalism as "grown-up children." To the extent that they respected the world of the whites the situation of the black slaves was exactly an infantile situation. This is also the situation of women in many civilizations; they can only submit to the laws, the gods, the customs, and the truths created by the males. Even today in western countries, among women who have not had in their work an apprenticeship of freedom, there are still many who take shelter in the shadow of men; they adopt without discussion the opinions and values recognized by their husband or their lover, and that allows them to develop childish qualities which are forbidden to adults because they are based on a feeling of irresponsibility. If what is called women's futility often has so much charm and grace, if it sometimes has a genuinely moving character, it is because it manifests a pure and gratuitous taste for existence, like the games of children; it is the absence of the serious. The unfortunate thing is that in many cases this thoughtlessness, this gaiety, these charming inventions imply a deep complicity with the world of men which they seem so graciously to be contesting, and it is a mistake to be astonished, once the structure which shelters them seems to be in danger, to see sensitive, ingenuous, and lightminded women show themselves harder, more bitter, and even more furious or cruel than their masters. It is then that we discover the difference which distinguishes them from an actual child: the child's situation is imposed upon him, whereas the woman (I mean the western woman of today) chooses it or at least consents to it. Ignorance and error are facts as inescapable as prison walls. The negro slave of the eighteenth century, the Mohammedan woman enclosed in a harem have no instrument, be it in thought or by astonishment or anger, which permits them to attack the civilization which oppresses them. Their behavior is defined and can be judged only within this given situation, and it is possible that in this situation, limited like every human situation, they realize a perfect assertion of their freedom. But once there appears a possibility of liberation, it is resignation of freedom not to exploit the possibility, a resignation which implies dishonesty and which is a positive fault.

The fact is that it is very rare for the infantile world to maintain itself beyond adolescence. From childhood on, flaws begin to be revealed in it. With astonishment, revolt and disrespect the child little by little asks himself, "Why must I act that way? What good is it? And what will happen if I act in another way?" He discovers his subjectivity; he discovers that of others. And when he arrives at the age of adolescence he begins to vacillate because he notices the contradictions among adults as well as their hesitations and weakness. Men stop appearing as if they were gods, and at the same time the adolescent discovers the human character of the reality about him. Language, customs, ethics, and values have their source in these uncertain creatures. The moment has come when he too is going to be called upon to participate in their operation; his acts weigh upon the earth as much as those of other men. He will have to choose and decide.

It is comprehensible that it is hard for him to live this moment of his history, and this is doubtless the deepest reason for the crisis of adolescence; the individual must at last assume his subjectivity.

From one point of view the collapsing of the serious world is a deliverance. Although he was irresponsible, the child also felt himself defenseless before obscure powers which directed the course of things. But whatever the joy of this liberation may be, it is not without great confusion that the adolescent finds himself cast into a world which is no longer ready-made, which has to be made; he is abandoned, unjustified, the prey of a freedom that is no longer chained up by anything. What will he do in the face of this new situation? This is the moment when he decides. If what might be called the natural history of an individual, his affective complexes, etcetera depend above all upon his childhood, it is adolescence which appears as the moment of moral choice. Freedom is then revealed and he must decide upon his attitude in the face of it. Doubtless, this decision can always be reconsidered, but the fact is that conversions are difficult because the world reflects back upon us a choice which is confirmed through this world which it has fashioned. Thus, a more and more rigorous circle is formed from which one is more and more unlikely to escape. Therefore, the misfortune which comes to man as a result of the fact that he was a child is that his freedom was first concealed from him and that all his life he will be nostalgic for the time when he did not know its exigencies.

This misfortune has still another aspect. Moral choice is free, and therefore unforeseeable. The child does not contain the man he will become. Yet, it is always on the basis of what he has been that a man decides upon what he wants to be. He draws the motivations of his moral attitude from within the character which he has given himself and from within the universe which is its correlative. Now, the child set up this character and this universe little by little, without foreseeing its development. He was ignorant of the disturbing aspect of this freedom which he was heedlessly exercising. He tranquilly abandoned himself to whims, laughter, tears, and anger which seemed to him to have no morrow and no danger, and yet which left ineffaceable imprints about him. The drama of original choice is that it goes on moment by moment for an entire lifetime, that it occurs without reason, before any reason, that freedom is there as if it were present only in the form of contingency. This contingency recalls, in a way, the arbitrariness of the grace distributed by God in Calvinistic doctrine. Here too there is a sort of predestination issuing not from an external tyranny but from the operation of the subject itself. Only, we think that man has always a possible recourse to himself. There is no choice so unfortunate that he cannot be saved.

It is in this moment of justification – a moment which extends throughout his whole adult life – that the attitude of man is placed on a moral plane. The contingent spontaneity can not be judged in the name of freedom. Yet a child already arouses sympathy or antipathy.

Every man casts himself into the world by making himself a lack of being; he thereby contributes to reinvesting it with human signification. He discloses it. And in this movement even the most outcast sometimes feel the joy of existing. They then manifest existence as a happiness and the world as a source of joy. But it is up to each one to make himself a lack of more or less various, profound, and rich aspects of being. What is called vitality, sensitivity, and intelligence are not ready-made qualities, but a way of casting oneself into the world and of disclosing being. Doubtless, every one casts himself into it on the basis of his physiological possibilities, but the body itself is not a brute fact. It expresses our relationship to the world, and that is why it is an object of sympathy or repulsion. And on the other hand, it determines no behavior. There is vitality only by means of free generosity. Intelligence supposes good will, and, inversely, a man is never stupid if he adapts his language and his behavior to his capacities, and sensitivity is nothing else but the presence which is attentive to the world and to itself. The reward for these spontaneous qualities issues from the fact that they make significances and goals appear in the world. They discover reasons for existing. They confirm us in the pride and joy of our destiny as man. To the extent that they subsist in an individual they still arouse sympathy, even if he has made himself hateful by the meaning which he has given to his life. I have heard it said that at the Nuremberg trial Goering exerted a certain seductive power on his judges because of the vitality which emanated from him.

If we were to try to establish a kind of hierarchy among men, we would put those who are denuded of this living warmth – the tepidity which the Gospel speaks of – on the lowest rung of the ladder. To exist is *to make oneself* a lack of being; it is to *cast* oneself into the world. Those who occupy themselves in restraining this original movement can be considered as sub-men. They have eyes and ears, but from their childhood on they make themselves blind and deaf, without love and without desire. This apathy manifests a fundamental fear in the face of existence, in the face of the risks and tensions which it implies. The sub-man rejects this "passion" which is his human condition, the laceration and the failure of that drive toward being which always misses its goal, but which thereby is the very existence which he rejects.

Such a choice immediately confirms itself. Just as a bad painter, by a single movement, paints bad paintings and is satisfied with them, whereas in a work of value the artist immediately recognizes the demand of a higher sort of work, in like fashion the original poverty of his project exempts the sub-man from seeking to legitimize it. He discovers around him only an insignificant and dull world. How could this naked world arouse within him any desire to feel, to understand, to live? The less he exists, the less is there reason for him to exist, since these reasons are created only by existing.

Yet, he exists. By the fact of transcending himself he indicates certain goals, he circumscribes certain values. But he at once effaces these uncertain shadows. His whole behavior tends toward an elimination of their ends. By the incoherence of his plans, by his haphazard whims, or by his indifference, he reduces to nothingness the meaning of his surpassing. His acts are never positive choices, only flights. He can not prevent himself from being a presence in the world, but he maintains this presence on the plane of bare facticity. However, if a man were permitted to be a brute fact, he would merge with the trees and pebbles which are not aware that they exist; we would consider these opaque lives with indifference. But the sub-man arouses contempt, that is, one recognizes him to be responsible for himself at the moment that one accuses him of not willing himself. – The fact is that no man is a datum which is passively suffered; the rejection of existence is still another way of existing; nobody can know the peace of the tomb while he is alive. There we have the defeat of the sub-man. He would like to forget himself, to be ignorant of himself, but the nothingness which is at the heart of man is also the consciousness that he has of himself. His negativity is revealed positively as anguish, desire, appeal, laceration, but as for the genuine return to the positive, the sub-man eludes it. He is afraid of engaging himself in a project as he is afraid of being disengaged and thereby of being in a state of danger before the future, in the midst of its possibilities. He is thereby led to take refuge in the ready-made values of the serious world. He will proclaim certain opinions; he will take shelter behind a label; and to hide his indifference he will readily abandon himself to verbal outbursts or even physical violence. One day, a monarchist, the next day, an anarchist, he is more readily anti-semitic, anti-clerical, or anti-republican. Thus, though we have defined him as a denial and a flight, the sub-man is not a harmless creature. He realizes himself in the world as a blind uncontrolled force which anybody can get control of. In lynchings, in pogroms, in all the great bloody movements organized by the fanaticism of seriousness and passion, movements where there is no risk, those who do the actual dirty work are recruited from among the sub-men. That is why every man who wills himself free within a human world fashioned by free men will be so disgusted by the sub-men. Ethics is the triumph of freedom over facticity, and the sub-man feels only the facticity of his existence. Instead of aggrandizing the reign of the human, he opposes his inert resistance to the projects of other men. No project has meaning in the world disclosed by such an existence. Man is defined as a wild flight. The world about him is bare and incoherent. Nothing ever happens; nothing merits desire or effort. The sub-man makes his way across a world deprived of meaning toward a death which merely confirms his long negation of himself. The only thing revealed in this experience is the absurd facticity of an existence which remains forever unjustified if it has not known how to justify itself. The sub-man experiences the desert of the world in his boredom. And the strange character of a universe with which he has created no bond also arouses fear in him. Weighted down by present events, he is bewildered before the darkness of the future which is haunted by frightful specters, war, sickness, revolution, fascism, bolshevism. The more indistinct these dangers are, the more fearful they become. The sub-man is not very clear about what he has to lose, since he has nothing, but this very uncertainty re-enforces his terror. Indeed, what he fears is that the shock of the unforeseen may remind him of the agonizing consciousness of himself.

Thus, fundamental as a man's fear in the face of existence may be, though he has chosen from his earliest years to deny his presence in the world, he can not keep himself from existing, he can not efface the agonizing evidence of his freedom. That is why, as we have just seen, in order to get rid of his freedom, he is led to engage it positively. The attitude of the sub-man passes logically over into that of the serious man; he forces himself to submerge his freedom in the content which the latter accepts from society. He loses himself in the object in order to annihilate his subjectivity. This certitude has been described so frequently that it will not be necessary to consider it at length. Hegel has spoken of it ironically. In *The Phenomenology of Mind* he has shown that the sub-man plays the part of the inessential in the face of the object which is considered as the essential. He suppresses himself to the advantage of the Thing, which, sanctified by respect, appears in the form of a Cause, science, philosophy, revolution, etc. But the truth is that this ruse miscarries, for the Cause can not save the individual insofar as he is a concrete and separate existence. After Hegel, Kierkegaard and Nietzsche also railed at the deceitful stupidity of the serious man and his universe. And *Being and Nothingness* is in large part a description of the serious man and his universe. The serious man gets rid of his freedom by claiming to subordinate it to values which would be unconditioned. He imagines that the accession to these values likewise permanently confers value upon himself. Shielded with "rights," he fulfills himself as a *being* who is escaping from the stress of existence. The serious is not defined by the nature of the ends pursued. A frivolous lady of fashion can have this mentality of the serious as well as an engineer. There is the serious from the moment that freedom denies itself to the advantage of ends which one claims are absolute.

Since all of this is well known, I should like to make only a few remarks in this place. It is easily understood why, of all the attitudes which are not genuine, the latter is the most widespread; because every man was first a child. After having lived under the eyes of the gods, having been given the promise of divinity, one does not readily accept becoming simply a man with all his anxiety and doubt. What is to be done? What is to be believed? Often the young man, who has not, like the sub-man, first rejected existence, so that these questions are not even raised, is nevertheless frightened at having to answer them. After a more or less long crisis, either he turns back toward the world of his parents and teachers or he adheres to the values which are new but seem to him just as sure. Instead of assuming an affectivity which would throw him dangerously beyond himself, he represses it. Liquidation, in its classic form of transference and sublimation, is the passage from the affective to the serious in the propitious shadow of dishonesty. The thing that matters to the serious man is not so much the nature of the object which he prefers to himself, but rather the fact of being able to lose himself in it. So much so, that the movement toward the object is, in fact, through his arbitrary act the most radical assertion of subjectivity: to believe for belief's sake, to will for will's sake is, detaching transcendence from its end, to realize one's freedom in its empty and absurd form of freedom of indifference.

The serious man's dishonesty issues from his being obliged ceaselessly to renew the denial of this freedom. He chooses to live in an infantile world, but to the child the values are really given. The serious man must mask the movement by which he gives them to himself, like the mythomaniac who while reading a love-letter pretends to forget that she has sent it to herself. We have already pointed out that certain adults can live in the universe of the serious in all honesty, for example, those who are denied all instruments of escape, those who are enslaved or who are mystified. The less economic and social circumstances allow an individual to act upon the world, the more this world appears to him as given. This is the case of women who inherit a long tradition of submission and of those who are called "the humble." There is often laziness and timidity in their resignation; their honesty is not quite complete; but to the extent that it. exists, their freedom remains available, it is not denied. They can, in their situation of ignorant and powerless individuals, know the truth of existence and raise themselves to a properly moral life. It even happens that they turn the freedom which they have thus won against the very object of their respect; thus, in *A Doll's House,* the childlike naivete of the heroine leads her to rebel against the lie of the serious. On the contrary, the man who has the necessary instruments to escape this lie and who does not want to use them consumes his freedom in denying, them. He makes himself serious. He dissimulates his subjectivity under the shield of rights which emanate from the ethical universe recognized by him; he is no longer a man, but a father, a boss, a member of the Christian Church or the Communist Party.

If one denies the subjective tension of freedom one is evidently forbidding himself universally to will freedom in an indefinite movement. By virtue of the fact that he refuses to recognize that he is freely establishing the value of the end he sets up, the serious man makes himself the slave of that end. He forgets that every goal is at the same time a point of departure and that human freedom is the ultimate, the unique end to which man should destine himself. He accords an absolute meaning to the epithet *useful,* which, in truth, has no more meaning if taken by itself than the words *high, low, right,* and *left.* It simply designates a relationship and requires a complement: useful *for* this or that. The complement itself must be put into question, and, as we shall see later on, the whole problem of action is then raised.

But the serious man puts nothing into question. For the military man, the army is useful; for the colonial administrator, the highway; for the serious revolutionary, the revolution – army, highway, revolution, productions becoming inhuman idols to which one will not hesitate to sacrifice man himself. Therefore, the serious man is dangerous. It is natural that he makes himself a tyrant. Dishonestly ignoring the subjectivity of his choice, he pretends that the unconditioned value of the object is being asserted through him; and by the same token he also ignores the value of the subjectivity and the freedom of others, to such an extent that, sacrificing them to the thing, he persuades himself that what he sacrifices is nothing. The colonial administrator who has raised the highway to the stature of an idol will have no scruple about assuring its construction at the price of a great number of lives of the natives; for, what value has the life of a native who is incompetent, lazy, and clumsy when it comes to building highways? The serious leads to a fanaticism which is as formidable as the fanaticism of passion. It is the fanaticism of the Inquisition which does not hesitate to impose a credo, that is, an internal movement, by means of external constraints. It is the fanaticism of the Vigilantes of America who defend morality by means of lynchings. It is the political fanaticism which empties politics of all human content and imposes the State, not *for* individuals, but *against* them.

In order to justify the contradictory, absurd, and outrageous aspects of this kind of behavior, the serious man readily takes refuge in disputing the serious, but it is the serious of others which he disputes, not his own. Thus, the colonial administrator is not unaware of the trick of irony. He contests the importance of the happiness, the comfort, the very life of the native, but he reveres the Highway, the Economy, the French Empire; he reveres himself as a servant of these divinities. Almost all serious men cultivate an expedient levity; we are familiar with the genuine gaiety of Catholics, the fascist "sense of humor." There are also some who do not even feel the need for such a weapon. They hide from themselves the incoherence of their choice by taking flight. As soon as the Idol is no longer concerned, the serious man slips into the attitude of the sub-man. He keeps himself from existing because he is not capable of existing without a guarantee. Proust observed with astonishment that a great doctor or a great professor often shows himself, outside of his specialty, to be lacking in sensitivity, intelligence, and humanity. The reason for this is that having abdicated his freedom, he has nothing else left but his techniques. In domains where his techniques are not applicable, he either adheres to the most ordinary of values or fulfills himself as a flight. The serious man stubbornly engulfs his transcendence in the object which bars the horizon and bolts the sky. The rest of the world is a faceless desert. Here again one sees how such a choice is immediately confirmed. If there is being only, for example, in the form of the Army, how could the military man wish for anything else than to multiply barracks and maneuvers? No appeal rises from the abandoned zones where nothing can be reaped because nothing has been sown. As soon as he leaves the staff, the old general becomes dull. That is why the serious man's life loses all meaning if he finds himself cut off from his ends. Ordinarily, he does not put all his eggs into one basket, but if it happens that a failure or old age ruins all his justifications, then, unless there is a conversion, which is always possible, he no longer has any relief except in flight; ruined, dishonored, this important personage is now only a "has-been." He joins the sub-man, unless by suicide he once and for all puts an end to the agony of his freedom.

It is in a state of fear that the serious man feels this dependence upon the object; and the first of virtues, in his eyes, is prudence. He escapes the anguish of freedom only to fall into a state of preoccupation, of worry. Everything is a threat to him, since the thing which he has set up as an idol is an externality and is thus in relationship with the whole universe and consequently threatened by the whole universe; and since, despite all precautions, he will never be the master of this exterior world to which he has consented to submit, he will be instantly upset by the uncontrollable course of events.

He will always be saying that he is disappointed, for his wish to have the world harden into a thing is belied by the very movement of life. The future will contest his present successes; his children will disobey him, his will will be opposed by those of strangers; he will be a prey to ill humor and bitterness. His very successes have a taste of ashes, for the serious is one of those ways of trying to realize the impossible synthesis of the in-itself and the for-itself. The serious man wills himself to be a god; but he is not one and knows it. He wishes to rid himself of his subjectivity, but it constantly risks being unmasked; it is unmasked. Transcending all goals, reflection wonders, "What's the use?" There then blazes forth the absurdity of a life which has sought outside of itself the justifications which it alone could give itself. Detached from the freedom which might have genuinely grounded them, all the ends that have been pursued appear arbitrary and useless.

This failure of the serious sometimes brings about a radical disorder. Conscious of being unable to be anything, man then decides to be nothing. We shall call this attitude nihilistic. The nihilist is close to the spirit of seriousness, for instead of realizing his negativity as a living movement, he conceives his annihilation in a substantial way. He wants to *be* nothing, and this nothing that he dreams of is still another sort of being, the exact Hegelian antithesis of being, a stationary datum. Nihilism is disappointed seriousness which has turned back upon itself. A choice of this kind is not encountered among those who, feeling the joy of existence, assume its gratuity. It appears either at the moment of adolescence, when the individual, seeing his child's universe flow away, feels the lack which is in his heart, or, later on, when the attempts to fulfill himself as a being have failed; in any case, among men who wish to rid themselves of the anxiety of their freedom by denying the world and themselves. By this rejection, they draw near to the sub-man. The difference is that their withdrawal is not their original movement. At first, they cast themselves into the world, sometimes even with a largeness of spirit. They exist and they know it.

It sometimes happens that, in his state of deception, a man maintains a sort of affection for the serious world; this is how Sartre describes Baudelaire in his study of the poet. Baudelaire felt a burning rancor in regard to the values of his childhood, but this rancor still involved some respect. Scorn alone liberated him. It was necessary for him that the universe which he rejected continue in order for him to detest it and scoff at it; it is the attitude of the demoniacal man as Jouhandeau has also described him: one stubbornly maintains the values of childhood, of a society, or of a Church in order to be able to trample upon them. The demoniacal man is still very close to the serious; he wants to believe in it; he confirms it by his very revolt; he feels himself as a negation and a freedom, but he does not realize this freedom as a positive liberation.

One can go much further in rejection by occupying himself not in scorning but in annihilating the rejected world and himself along with it. For example, the man who gives himself to a cause which he knows to be lost chooses to merge the world with one of its aspects which carries within it the germ of its ruin, involving himself in this condemned universe and condemning himself with it. Another man devotes his time and energy to an undertaking which was not doomed to failure at the start but which he himself is bent on ruining. Still another rejects each of his projects one after the other, frittering them away in a series of caprices and thereby systematically annulling the ends which he is aiming at. The constant negation of the word by the word, of the act by the act, of art by art was realized by Dadaist incoherence. By following a strict injunction to commit disorder and anarchy, one achieved the abolition of all behavior, and therefore of all ends and of oneself.

But this will to negation is forever belying itself, for it manifests itself as a presence at the very moment that it displays itself. It therefore implies a constant tension, inversely symmetrical with the existential and more painful tension, for if it is true that man is not, it is also true that he exists, and in order to realize his negativity positively he will have to contradict constantly the movement of existence. If one does not resign himself to suicide one slips easily into a more stable attitude than the shrill rejection of nihilism. Surrealism provides us with a historical and concrete example of different possible kinds of evolution. Certain initiates, such as Vache and Crevel, had recourse to the radical solution of suicide. Others destroyed their bodies and ruined their minds by drugs. Others succeeded in a sort of moral suicide; by dint of depopulating the world around them, they found themselves in a desert, with themselves reduced to the level of the sub-man; they no longer try to flee, they are fleeing. There are also some who have again sought out the security of the serious. They have reformed, arbitrarily choosing marriage, politics, or religion as refuges. Even the surrealists who have wanted to remain faithful to themselves have been unable to avoid returning to the positive, to the serious. The negation of aesthetic, spiritual, and moral values has become an ethics; unruliness has become a rule. We have been present at the establishment of a new Church, with its dogmas, its rites, its faithful, its priests, and even its martyrs; today, there is nothing of the destroyer in Breton; he is a pope. And as every assassination of painting is still a painting, a lot of surrealists have found themselves the authors of positive works; their revolt has become the matter on which their career has been built. Finally, some of them, in a genuine return to the positive, have been able to realize their freedom; they have given it a content without disavowing it. They have engaged themselves, without losing themselves, in political action, in intellectual or artistic research, in family or social life.

The attitude of the nihilist can perpetuate itself as such only if it reveals itself as a positivity at its very core. Rejecting his own existence, the nihilist must also reject the existences which confirm it. If he wills himself to be nothing, all mankind must also be annihilated; otherwise, by means of the presence of this world that the Other reveals he meets himself as a presence in the world. But this thirst for destruction immediately takes the form of a desire for power. The taste of nothingness joins the original taste of being whereby every man is first defined; he realizes himself as a being by making himself that by which nothingness comes into the world. Thus, Nazism was both a will for power and a will for suicide at the same time. From a historical point of view, Nazism has many other features besides; in particular, beside the dark romanticism which led Rauschning to entitle his work *The Revolution of Nihilism,* we also find a gloomy seriousness. The fact is that Nazism was in the service of petit bourgeois seriousness. But it is interesting to note that its ideology did not make this alliance impossible, for the serious often rallies to a partial nihilism, denying everything which is not its object in order to hide from itself the antinomies of action.

A rather pure example of this impassioned nihilism is the well-known case of Drieu la Rochelle. *The Empty Suitcase* is the testimony of a young man who acutely felt the fact of existing as a lack of being, of not being. This is a genuine experience on the basis of which the only possible salvation is to assume the lack, to side with the man who exists against the idea of a God who does not. On the contrary – a novel like *Gilles* is proof – Drieu stubbornly persisted in his deception. In his hatred of himself he chose to reject his condition as a man, and this led him to hate all men along with himself. Gilles knows satisfaction only when he fires on Spanish workers and sees the flow of blood which he compares to the redeeming blood of Christ; as if the only salvation by man were the death of other men, whereby perfect negation is achieved. It is natural that this path ended in collaboration, the ruin of a detested world being merged for Drieu with the annulment of himself. An external failure led him to give to his life a conclusion which it called for dialectically: suicide.

The nihilist attitude manifests a certain truth. In this attitude one experiences the ambiguity of the human condition. But the mistake is that it defines man not as the positive existence of a lack, but as a lack at the heart of existence, whereas the truth is that existence is not a lack as such. And if freedom is experienced in this case in the form of rejection, it is not genuinely fulfilled. The nihilist is right in thinking that the world *possesses* no justification and that he himself is nothing. But he forgets that it is up to him to justify the world and to man himself exist validly. Instead of integrating death into life, he sees in it the only truth of the life which appears to him as a disguised death. However, there is life, and the nihilist knows that he is alive. That's where his failure lies. He rejects existence without managing to eliminate it. He denies any meaning to his transcendence, and yet he transcends himself. A man who delights in freedom can find an ally in the nihilist because they contest the serious world together, but be also sees in him an enemy insofar as the nihilist is a systematic rejection of the world and man, and if this rejection ends up in a positive desire, destruction, it then establishes a tyranny which freedom must stand up against.

The fundamental fault of the nihilist is that, challenging all given values, he does not find, beyond their ruin, the importance of that universal, absolute end which freedom itself is. It is possible that, even in this failure, a man may nevertheless keep his taste for an existence which he originally felt as a joy. Hoping for no justification, he will nevertheless take delight in living. He will not turn aside from things which he does not believe in. He will seek a pretext in them for a gratuitous display of activity. Such a man is what is generally called an adventurer. He throws himself into his undertakings with zest, into exploration, conquest, war, speculation, love, politics, but he does not attach himself to the end at which he aims; only to his conquest. He likes action for its own sake. He finds joy in spreading through the world a freedom which remains indifferent to its content. Whether the taste for adventure appears to be based on nihilistic despair or whether it is born directly from the experience of the happy days of childhood, it always implies that freedom is realized as an independence in regard to the serious world and that, on the other hand, the ambiguity of existence is felt not as a lack but in its positive aspect. This attitude dialectically envelops nihilism's opposition to the serious and the opposition to nihilism by existence as such. But, of course, the concrete history of an individual does not necessarily espouse this dialectic, by virtue of the fact that his condition is wholly present to him at each moment and because his freedom before it is, at every moment, total. From the time of his adolescence a man can define himself as an adventurer. The union of an original, abundant vitality and a reflective scepticism will particularly lead to this choice.

It is obvious that this choice is very close to a genuinely moral attitude. The adventurer does not propose to be; he deliberately makes himself a lack of being; he aims expressly at existence; though engaged in his undertaking, he is at the same time detached from the goal. Whether he succeeds or fails, he goes right ahead throwing himself into a new enterprise to which he will give himself with the same indifferent ardor. It is not from things that he expects the justification of his choices. Considering such behavior at the moment of its subjectivity, we see that it conforms to the requirements of ethics, and if existentialism were solipsistic, as is generally claimed, it would have to regard the adventurer as its perfect hero.

First of all, it should be noticed that the adventurer's attitude is not always pure. Behind the appearance of caprice, there are many men who pursue a secret goal in utter seriousness; for example, fortune or glory. They proclaim their scepticism in regard to recognized values. They do not take politics seriously. They thereby allow themselves to be collaborationists in '41 and communists in '45, and it is true they don't give a hang about the interests of the French people or the proletariat; they are attached to their career, to their success. This *arrivisme* is at the very antipodes of the spirit of adventure, because the zest for existence is then never experienced in its gratuity. It also happens that the genuine love for adventure is inextricably mixed with an attachment to the values of the serious. Cortez and the conquistadors served God and the emperor by serving their own pleasure. Adventure can also be shot through with passion. The taste for conquest is often subtly tied up with the taste for possession. Was seduction all that Don Juan liked? Did he not also like women? Or was he not even looking for a woman capable of satisfying him?

But even if we consider adventure in its purity, it appears to us to be satisfying only at a subjective moment, which, in fact, is a quite abstract moment. The adventurer always meets others along the way; the conquistador meets the Indians; the condottiere hacks out a path through blood and ruins; the explorer has comrades about him or soldiers under his orders; every Don Juan is confronted with Elviras. Every undertaking unfolds in a human world and affects men. What distinguishes adventure from a simple game is that the adventurer does not limit himself to asserting his existence in solitary fashion. He asserts it in relationship to other existences. He has to declare himself.

Two attitudes are possible. He can become conscious of the real requirements of his own freedom, which can will itself only by destining itself to an open future, by seeking to extend itself by means of the freedom of others. Therefore, in any case, the freedom of other men must be respected and they must be helped to free themselves. Such a law imposes limits upon action and at the same time immediately gives it a content. Beyond the rejected seriousness is found a genuine seriousness. But the man who acts in this way, whose end is the liberation of himself and others, who forces himself to respect this end through the means which he uses to attain it, no longer deserves the name of adventurer. One would not dream for example, of applying it to a Lawrence, who was so concerned about the lives of his companions and the freedom of others, so tormented by the human problems which all action raises. One is then in the presence of a genuinely free man.

The man we call an adventurer, on the contrary, is one who remains indifferent to the content, that is, to the human meaning of his action, who thinks he can assert his own existence without taking into account that of others. The fate of Italy mattered very little to the Italian condottiere; the massacres of the Indians meant nothing to Pizarro; Don Juan was unaffected by Elvira's tears. Indifferent to the ends they set up for themselves, they were still more indifferent to the means of attaining them; they cared only for their pleasure or their glory. This implies that the adventurer shares the nihilist's contempt for men. And it is by this very contempt that he believes he breaks away from the contemptible condition in which those who do not imitate his pride are stagnating. Thus, nothing prevents him from sacrificing these insignificant beings to his own will for power. He will treat them like instruments; he will destroy them if they get in his way. But meanwhile he appears as an enemy in the eyes of others. His undertaking is not only an individual wager; it is a combat. He can not win the game without making himself a tyrant or a hangman. And as he can not impose this tyranny without help, he is obliged to serve the regime which will allow him to exercise it. He needs money, arms, soldiers, or the support of the police and the laws. It is not a matter of chance, but a dialectical necessity which leads the adventurer to be complacent regarding all regimes which defend the privilege of a class or a party, and more particularly authoritarian regimes and fascism. He needs fortune, leisure, and enjoyment, and he will take these goods as supreme ends in order to be prepared to remain free in regard to any end. Thus, confusing a quite external availability with real freedom, he falls, with a pretext of independence, into the servitude of the object. He will range himself on the side of the regimes which guarantee him his privileges, and he will prefer those which confirm him in his contempt regarding the common herd. He will make himself its accomplice, its servant, or even its valet, alienating a freedom which, in reality, can not confirm itself as such if it does not wear its own face. In order to have wanted to limit it to itself, in order to have emptied it of all concrete content, he realizes it only as an abstract independence which turns into servitude. He must submit to masters unless he makes himself the supreme master. Favorable circumstances are enough to transform the adventurer into a dictator. He carries the seed of one within him, since he regards mankind as indifferent matter destined to support the game of his existence. But what he then knows is the supreme servitude of tyranny.

Hegel's criticism of the tyrant is applicable to the adventurer to the extent that he is himself a tyrant, or at the very least an accomplice of the oppressor. No man can save himself alone. Doubtless, in the very heat of an action the adventurer can know a joy which is sufficient unto itself, but once the undertaking is over and has congealed behind him into a thing, it must, in order to remain alive, be animated anew by a human intention which must transcend it toward the future into recognition or admiration. When he dies, the adventurer will be surrendering his whole life into the hands of men; the only meaning it will have will be the one they confer upon it. He knows this since he talks about himself, often in books. For want of a work, many desire to bequeath their own personality to posterity: at least during their lifetime they need the approval of a few faithful. Forgotten and detested, the adventurer loses the taste for his own existence. Perhaps without his knowing it, it seems so precious to him because of others. It willed itself to be an affirmation, an example to all mankind. Once it falls back upon itself, it becomes futile and unjustified.

Thus, the adventurer devises a sort of moral behavior because he assumes his subjectivity positively. But if he dishonestly refuses to recognize that this subjectivity necessarily transcends itself toward others, he will enclose himself in a false independence which will indeed be servitude. To the free man he will be only a chance ally in whom one can have no confidence; he will easily become an enemy. His fault is believing that one can do something for oneself without others and even against them.

The passionate man is, in a way, the antithesis of the adventurer. In him too there is a sketch of the synthesis of freedom and its content. But in the adventurer it is the content which does not succeed in being genuinely fulfilled. Whereas in the passionate man it is subjectivity which fails to fulfill itself genuinely.

What characterizes the passionate man is that he sets up the object as an absolute, not, like the serious man, as a thing detached from himself, but as a thing disclosed by his subjectivity. There are transitions between the serious and passion. A goal which was first willed in the name of the serious can become an object of passion; inversely, a passionate attachment can wither into a serious relationship. But real passion asserts the subjectivity of its involvement. In amorous passion particularly, one does not want the beloved being to be admired objectively; one prefers to think her unknown, unrecognized; the lover thinks that his appropriation of her is greater if he is alone in revealing her worth. That is the genuine thing offered by all passion. The moment of subjectivity therein vividly asserts itself, in its positive form, in a movement toward the object. It is only when passion has been degraded to an organic need that it ceases to choose itself. But as long as it remains alive it does so because subjectivity is animating it; if not pride, at least complacency and obstinacy. At the same time that it is an assumption of this subjectivity, it is also a disclosure of being. It helps populate the world with desirable objects, with exciting meanings. However, in the passions which we shall call maniacal, to distinguish them from the generous passions, freedom does not find its genuine form. The passionate man seeks possession; he seeks to attain being. The failure and the hell which he creates for himself have been described often enough. He causes certain rare treasures to appear in the world, but he also depopulates it. Nothing exists outside of his stubborn project; therefore nothing can induce him to modify his choices. And having involved his whole life with an external object which can continually escape him, he tragically feels his dependence. Even if it does not definitely disappear, the object never gives itself. The passionate man makes himself a lack of being not that there might *be* being, but in order to be. And he remains at a distance; he is never fulfilled.

That is why though the passionate man inspires a certain admiration, he also inspires a kind of horror at the same time. One admires the pride of a subjectivity which chooses its end without bending itself to any foreign law and the precious brilliance of the object revealed by the force of this assertion. But one also considers the solitude in which this subjectivity encloses itself as injurious. Having withdrawn into an unusual region of the world, seeking not to communicate with other men, this freedom is realized only as a separation. Any conversation, any relationship with the passionate man is impossible. In the eyes of those who desire a communion of freedom, he therefore appears as a stranger, an obstacle. He opposes an opaque resistance to the movement of freedom which wills itself infinite. The passionate man is not only an inert facticity. He too is on the way to tyranny. He knows that his will emanates only from him, but he can nevertheless attempt to impose it upon others. He authorizes himself to do that by a partial nihilism. Only the object of his passion appears real and full to him. All the rest are insignificant. Why not betray, kill, grow violent? It is never *nothing* that one destroys. The whole universe is perceived only as an ensemble of means or obstacles through which it is a matter of attaining the thing in which one has engaged his being. Not intending his freedom for men, the passionate man does not recognize them as freedoms either. He will not hesitate to treat them as things. If the object of his passion concerns the world in general, this tyranny becomes fanaticism. In all fanatical movements there exists an element of the serious. The values invented by certain men in a passion of hatred, fear, or faith are thought and willed by others as given realities. But there is no serious fanaticism which does not have a passional base, since all adhesion to the serious world is brought about by repressed tendencies and complexes. Thus, maniacal passion represents a damnation for the one who chooses it, and for other men it is one of the forms of separation which disunites freedoms. It leads to struggle and oppression. A man who seeks being far from other men, seeks it against them at the same time that he loses himself.

Yet, a conversion can start within passion itself. The cause of the passionate man's torment is his distance from the object; but he must accept it instead of trying to eliminate it. It is the condition within which the object is disclosed. The individual will then find his joy in the very wrench which separates him from the being of which he makes himself a lack. Thus, in the letters of Mademoiselle de Lespinasse there is constant passing from grief to the assumption of this grief. The lover describes her tears and her tortures, but she asserts that she loves this unhappiness. It is also a source of delight for her. She likes the other to appear as another through her separation. It pleases her to exalt, by her very suffering, that strange existence which she chooses to set up as worthy of any sacrifice. It is only as something strange, forbidden, as something free, that the other is revealed as an other. And to love him genuinely is to love him in his otherness and in that freedom by which he escapes. Love is then renunciation of all possession, of all confusion. One renounces being in order that there may be that being which one is not. Such generosity, moreover, can not be exercised on behalf of any object whatsoever. One can not love a pure thing in its independence and its separation, for the thing does not have positive independence. If a man prefers the land he has discovered to the possession of this land, a painting or a statue to their material presence, it is insofar as they appear to him as possibilities open to other men. Passion is converted to genuine freedom only if one destines his existence to other existences through the being – whether thing or man – at which he aims, without hoping to entrap it in the destiny of the in-itself.

Thus, we see that no existence can be validly fulfilled if it is limited to itself. It appeals to the existence of others. The idea of such a dependence is frightening, and the separation and multiplicity of existants raises highly disturbing problems. One can understand that men who are aware of the risks and the inevitable element of failure involved in any engagement in the world attempt to fulfill themselves outside of the world. Man is permitted to separate himself from this world by contemplation, to think about it, to create it anew. Some men, instead of building their existence upon the indefinite unfolding of time, propose to assert it in its eternal aspect and to achieve it as an absolute. They hope, thereby, to surmount the ambiguity of their condition. Thus, many intellectuals seek their salvation either in critical thought or creative activity.

We have seen that the serious contradicts itself by the fact that not everything can be taken seriously. It slips into a partial nihilism. But nihilism is unstable. It tends to return to the positive. Critical thought attempts to militate everywhere against all aspects of the serious but without foundering in the anguish of pure negation. It sets up a superior, universal, and timeless value, objective truth. And, correlatively, the critic defines himself positively as the independence of the mind. Crystallizing the negative movement of the criticism of values into a positive reality, he also crystallizes the negativity proper to all mind into a positive presence. Thus, he thinks that he himself escapes all earthly criticism. He does not have to choose between the highway and the native, between America and Russia, between production and freedom. He understands, dominates, and rejects, in the name of total truth, the necessarily partial truths which every human engagement discloses. But ambiguity is at the heart of his very attitude, for the independent man is still a man with his particular situation in the world, and what he defines as objective truth is the object of his own choice. His criticisms fall into the world of particular men. He does not merely describe. He takes sides. If he does not assume the subjectivity of his judgment, he is inevitably caught in the trap of the serious. Instead of the independent mind he claims to be, he is only the shameful servant of a cause to which he has not chosen to rally.

The artist and the writer force themselves to surmount existence in another way. They attempt to realize it as an absolute. What makes their effort genuine is that they do not propose to attain being. They distinguish themselves thereby from an engineer or a maniac. It is existence which they are trying to pin down and make eternal. The word, the stroke, the very marble indicate the object insofar as it is an absence. Only, in the work of art the lack of being returns to the positive. Time is stopped, clear forms and finished meanings rise up. In this return, existence is confirmed and establishes its own justification. This is what Kant said when he defined art as "a finality without end." By virtue of the fact that he has thus set up an absolute object, the creator is then tempted to consider himself as absolute. He justifies the world and therefore thinks he has no need of anyone to justify himself. If the work becomes an idol whereby the artist thinks that he is fulfilling himself as being, he is closing himself up in the universe of the serious; he is falling into the illusion which Hegel exposed when he described the race of "intellectual animals."

There is no way for a man to escape from this world. It is in this world that – avoiding the pitfalls we have just pointed out – he must realize himself morally. Freedom must project itself toward its own reality through a content whose value it establishes. An end is valid only by a return to the freedom which established it and which willed itself through this end. But this will implies that freedom is not to be engulfed in any goal; neither is it to dissipate itself vainly without aiming at a goal. It is not necessary for the subject to seek to be, but it must desire that there *be* being. To will oneself free and to will that there be *being* are one and the same choice, the choice that man makes of himself as a presence in the world. We can neither say that the free man wants freedom in order to desire being, nor that he wants the disclosure of being by freedom. These are two aspects of a single reality. And whichever be the one under consideration, they both imply the bond of each man with all others.

This bond does not immediately reveal itself to everybody. A young man wills himself free. He wills that there be being. This spontaneous liberality which casts him ardently into the world can ally itself to what is commonly called egoism. Often the young man perceives only that aspect of his relationship to others whereby others appear as enemies. In the preface to *The Inner Experience* Georges Bataille emphasizes very forcefully that each individual wants to be All. He sees in every other man and particularly in those whose existence is asserted with most brilliance, a limit, a condemnation of himself. "Each consciousness," said Hegel, "seeks the death of the other." And indeed at every moment others are stealing the whole world away from me. The first movement is to hate them.

But this hatred is naive, and the desire immediately struggles against itself. If I were really everything there would be nothing beside me; the world would be empty. There would be nothing to possess, and I myself would be nothing. If he is reasonable, the young man immediately understands that by taking the world away from me, others also give it to me, since a thing is given to me only by the movement which snatches it from me. To will that there be being is also to will that there be men by and for whom the world is endowed with human significations. One can reveal the world only on a basis revealed by other men. No project can be defined except by its interference with other projects. To make being "be" is to communicate with others by means of being.

This truth is found in another form when we say that freedom can not will itself without aiming at an open future. The ends which it gives itself must be unable to be transcended by any reflection, but only the freedom of other men can extend them beyond our life. I have tried to show in *Pyrrhus and Cineas* that every man needs the freedom of other men and, in a sense, always wants it, even though he may be a tyrant; the only thing he fails to do is to assume honestly the consequences of such a wish. Only the freedom of others keeps each one of us from hardening in the absurdity of facticity. And if we are to believe the Christian myth of creation, God himself was in agreement on this point with the existentialist doctrine since, in the words of an anti-fascist priest, "He had such respect for man that He created him free."

Thus, it can be seen to what an extent those people are mistaken – or are lying – who try to make of existentialism a solipsism, like Nietzsche, would exalt the bare will to power. According to this interpretation, as widespread as it is erroneous, the individual, knowing himself and choosing himself as the creator of his own values, would seek to impose them on others. The result would be a conflict of opposed wills enclosed in their solitude. But we have seen that, on the contrary, to the extent that passion, pride, and the spirit of adventure lead to this tyranny and its conflicts, existentialist ethics condemns them; and it does so not in the name of an abstract law, but because, if it is true that every project emanates from subjectivity, it is also true that this subjective movement establishes by itself a surpassing of subjectivity. Man can find a justification of his own existence only in the existence of other men. Now, he needs such a justification; there is no escaping it. Moral anxiety does not come to man from without; he finds within himself the anxious question, "What's the use?" Or, to put it better, he himself is this urgent interrogation. He flees it only by fleeing himself, and as soon as he exists he answers. It may perhaps be said that it is for himself that he is moral, and that such an attitude is egotistical. But there is no ethics against which this charge, which immediately destroys itself, can not be leveled; for how can I worry about what does not concern me? I concern others and they concern me. There we have an irreducible truth. The me-others relationship is as indissoluble as the subject-object relationship.

At the same time the other charge which is often directed at existentialism also collapses: of being a formal doctrine, incapable of proposing any content to the freedom which it wants engaged. To will oneself free is also to will others free. This will is not an abstract formula. It points out to each person concrete action to be achieved. But the others are separate, even opposed, and the man of good will sees concrete and difficult problems arising in his relations with them. It is this positive aspect of morality that we are now going to examine.

III The Positive Aspect of Ambiguity

1. <u>The Aesthetic Attitude</u>
2. <u>Freedom and Liberation</u>
3. <u>The Antinomies of Action</u>
4. <u>The Present and the Future</u>
5. <u>Ambiguity</u>

The Aesthetic Attitude

Thus, every man has to do with other men. The world in which he engages himself is a human world in which each object is penetrated with human meanings. It is a speaking world from which solicitations and appeals rise up. This means that, through this world, each individual can give his freedom a concrete content. He must disclose the world with the purpose of further disclosure and by the same movement try to free men, by means of whom the world takes on meaning. But we shall find here the same objection that we met when we examined the abstract moment of individual ethics. If every man is free, he can not *will* himself free. Likewise the objection will be raised that he can will nothing for another since that other is free in all circumstances; men are always disclosing being, in Buchenwald as well as in the blue isles of the Pacific, in hovels as well as in palaces; something is always happening in the world, and in the movement of keeping being at a distance, can one not consider its different transformations with a detached joy, or find reasons for acting? No solution is better or worse than any other.

We may call this attitude aesthetic because the one who adopts it claims to have no other relation with the world than that of detached contemplation; outside of time, and far from men, he faces history, which he thinks he does not belong to, like a pure beholding; this impersonal version equalizes all situations; it apprehends them only in the indifference of their differences; it excludes any preference.

Thus, the lover of historical works is present at the birth and the downfall of Athens, Rome, and Byzantium with the same serene passion. The tourist considers the arena of the Coliseum, the Latifundia of Syracuse, the thermal baths, the palaces, the temples, the prisons, and the churches with the same tranquil curiosity: these things existed, that is enough to satisfy him. Why not also consider with impartial interest those that exist today? One finds this temptation among many Italians who are weighed down by a magical and deceptive past; the present already seems to them like a future past. Wars, civil disputes, invasions and slavery have succeeded one another in their land. Each moment of that tormented history is contradicted by the following one; and yet in the very midst of this vain agitation there arose domes, statues, bas-reliefs, paintings and palaces which have remained intact through the centuries and which still enchant the men of today. One can imagine an intellectual Florentine being skeptical about the great uncertain movements which are stirring up his country and which will die out as did the seethings of the centuries which have gone by: as he sees it, the important thing is merely to understand the temporary events and through them to cultivate that beauty which perishes not. Many Frenchmen also sought relief in this thought in 1940 and the years which followed. "Let's try to take the point of view of history," they said upon learning that the Germans had entered Paris. And during the whole occupation certain intellectuals sought to keep "aloof from the fray" and to consider impartially contingent facts which did not concern them.

But we note at once that such an attitude appears in moments of discouragement and confusion; in fact, it is a position of withdrawal, a way of fleeing the truth of the present. As concerns the past, this eclecticism is legitimate; we are no longer in a live situation in regard to Athens, Sparta, or Alexandria, and the very idea of a choice has no meaning. But the present is not a potential past; it is the moment of choice and action; we can not avoid living it through a project; and there is no project which is purely contemplative since one always projects himself toward something, toward the future; to put oneself "outside" is still a way of living the inescapable fact that one is inside; those French intellectuals who, in the name of history, poetry, or art, sought to rise above the drama of the age, were willy-nilly its actors more or less explicitly, they were playing the occupier's game. Likewise, the Italian aesthete, occupied in caressing the marbles and bronzes of Florence, is playing a political role in the life of his country by his very inertia. One can not justify all that is by asserting that everything may equally be the object of contemplation, since man never contemplates: he does.

It is for the artist and the writer that the problem is raised in a particularly acute and at the same time equivocal manner, for then one seeks to set up the indifference of human situations not in the name of pure contemplation, but of a definite project: the creator projects toward the work of art a subject which he justifies insofar as it is the matter of this work; any subject may thus be admitted, a massacre as well as a masquerade. This aesthetic justification is sometimes so striking that it betrays the author's aim; let us say that a writer wants to communicate the horror inspired in him by children working in sweatshops; he produces so beautiful a book that, enchanted by the tale, the style, and the images, we forget the horror of the sweatshops or even start admiring it. Will we not then be inclined to think that if death, misery, and injustice can be transfigured for our delight, it is not an evil for there to be death, misery, and injustice?

But here too we must not confuse the present with the past. With regard to the past, no further action is possible. There have been war, plague, scandal, and treason, and there is no way of our preventing their having taken place; the executioner became an executioner and the victim underwent his fate as a victim without us; all that we can do is to reveal it, to integrate it into the human heritage, to raise it to the dignity of the aesthetic existence which bears within itself its finality; but first this history had to occur: it occurred as scandal, revolt, crime, or sacrifice, and we were able to try to save it only because it first offered us a form. Today must also exist before being confirmed in its existence: its destination in such a way that everything about it already seemed justified and that there was no more of it to reject, then there would also be nothing to say about it, for no form would take shape in it; it is revealed only through rejection, desire, hate and love. In order for the artist to have a world to express he must first be situated in this world, oppressed or oppressing, resigned or rebellious, a man among men. But at the heart of his existence he finds the exigency which is common to all men; he must first will freedom within himself and universally; he must try to conquer it: in the light of this project situations are graded and reasons for acting are made manifest.

Freedom and Liberation

One of the chief objections leveled against existentialism is that the precept "to will freedom" is only a hollow formula and offers no concrete content for action. But that is because one has begun by emptying the word freedom of its concrete meaning; we have already seen that freedom realizes itself only by engaging itself in the world: to such an extent that man's project toward freedom is embodied for him in definite acts of behavior.

To will freedom and to will to disclose being are one and the same choice; hence, freedom takes a positive and constructive step which causes being to pass to existence in a movement which is constantly surpassed. Science, technics, art, and philosophy are indefinite conquests of existence over being; it is by assuming themselves as such that they take on their genuine aspect; it is in the light of this assumption that the word progress finds its veridical meaning. It is not a matter of approaching a fixed limit: absolute Knowledge or the happiness of man or the perfection of beauty; all human effort would then be doomed to failure, for with each step forward the horizon recedes a step; for man it is a matter of pursuing the expansion of his existence and of retrieving this very effort as an absolute.

Science condemns itself to failure when, yielding to the infatuation of the serious, it aspires to attain being, to contain it, and to possess it; but it finds its truth if it considers itself as a free engagement of thought in the given, aiming, at each discovery, not at fusion with the thing, but at the possibility of new discoveries; what the mind then projects is the concrete accomplishment of its freedom. The attempt is sometimes made to find an objective justification of science in technics; but ordinarily the mathematician is concerned with mathematics and the physicist with physics, and not with their applications. And, furthermore, technics itself is not objectively justified; if it sets up as absolute goals the saving of time and work which it enables us to realize and the comfort and luxury which it enables us to have access to, then it appears useless and absurd, for the time that one gains can not be accumulated in a store house; it is contradictory to want to save up existence, which, the fact is, exists only by being spent, and there is a good case for showing that airplanes, machines, the telephone, and the radio do not make men of today happier than those of former times. But actually it is not a question of giving men time and happiness, it is not a question of stopping the movement of life: it is a question of fulfilling it. If technics is attempting to make up for this lack, which is at the very heart of existence, it fails radically; but it escapes all criticism if one admits that, through it, existence, far from wishing to repose in the security of being, thrusts itself ahead of itself in order to thrust itself still farther ahead, that it aims at an indefinite disclosure of being by the transformation of the thing into an instrument and at the opening of ever new possibilities for man. As for art, we have already said that it should not attempt to set up idols; it should reveal existence as a reason for existing; that is really why Plato, who wanted to wrest man away from the earth and assign him to the heaven of Ideas, condemned the poets; that is why every humanism on the other hand, crowns them with laurels. Art reveals the transitory as an absolute; and as the transitory existence is perpetuated through the centuries, art too, through the centuries, must perpetuate this never-to-be-finished revelation. Thus, the constructive activities of man take on a valid meaning only when they are assumed as a movement toward freedom; and reciprocally, one sees that such a movement is concrete: discoveries, inventions, industries, culture, paintings, and books people the world concretely and open concrete possibilities to men.

Perhaps it is permissible to dream of a future when men will know no other use of their freedom than this free unfurling of itself; constructive activity would be possible for all; each one would be able to aim positively through his projects at his own future. But today the fact is that there are men who can justify their life only by a negative action. As we have already seen, every man transcends himself. But it happens that this transcendence is condemned to fall uselessly back upon itself because it is cut off from its goals. That is what defines a situation of oppression. Such a situation is never natural: man is never oppressed by things; in any case, unless he is a naive child who hits stones or a mad prince who orders the sea to be thrashed, he does not rebel against things, but only against other men. The resistance of the thing sustains the action of man as air sustains the flight of the dove; and by projecting himself through it man accepts its being an obstacle; he assumes the risk of a setback in which he does not see a denial of his freedom. The explorer knows that he may be forced to withdraw before arriving at his goal; the scientist, that a certain phenomenon may remain obscure to him; the technician, that his attempt may prove abortive: these withdrawals and errors are another way of disclosing the world. Certainly, a material obstacle may cruelly stand in the way of an undertaking: floods, earthquakes, grasshoppers, epidemics and plague are scourges; but here we have one of the truths of Stoicism: a man must assume even these misfortunes, and since he must never resign himself in favor of any *thing,* no destruction of a thing will ever be a radical ruin for him; even his death is not an evil since he is man only insofar as he is mortal: he must assume it as the natural limit of his life, as the risk implied by every step. Only man can be an enemy for man; only he can rob him of the meaning of his acts and his life because it also belongs only to him alone to confirm it in its existence, to recognize it in actual fact as a freedom. It is here that the Stoic distinction between "things which do not depend upon us" and those which "depend upon us" proves to be insufficient: for "we" is legion and not an individual; each one depends upon others, and what happens to me by means of others depends upon me as regards its meaning; one does not submit to a war or an occupation as he does to an earthquake: he must take sides for or against, and the foreign wills thereby become allied or hostile. It is this interdependence which explains why oppression is possible and why it is hateful. As we have seen, my freedom, in order to fulfill itself, requires that it emerge into an open future: it is other men who open the future to me, it is they who, setting up the world of tomorrow, define my future; but if, instead of allowing me to participate in this constructive movement, they oblige me to consume my transcendence in vain, if they keep me below the level which they have conquered and on the basis of which new conquests will be achieved then they are cutting me off from the future, they are changing me into a thing. Life is occupied in both perpetuating itself and in surpassing itself; if all it does is maintain itself, then living is only not dying, and human existence is indistinguishable from an absurd vegetation; a life justifies itself only if its effort to perpetuate itself is integrated into its surpassing and if this surpassing has no other limits than those which the subject assigns himself. Oppression divides the world into two clans: those who enlighten mankind by thrusting it ahead of itself and those who are condemned to mark time hopelessly in order merely to support the collectivity; their life is a pure repetition of mechanical gestures; their leisure is just about sufficient for them to regain their strength; the oppressor feeds himself on their transcendence and refuses to extend it by a free recognition. The oppressed has only one solution: to deny the harmony of that mankind from which an attempt is made to exclude him, to prove that he is a man and that he is free by revolting against the tyrants. In order to prevent this revolt, one of the ruses of oppression is to camouflage itself behind a natural situation since, after all, one can not revolt against nature. When a conservative wishes to show that the proletariat is not oppressed, he declares that the present distribution of wealth is a natural fact and that there is thus no means of rejecting it; and doubtless he has a good case for proving that, strictly speaking, he is not *stealing* from the worker "the product of his labor," since the word *theft* supposes social conventions which in other respects authorizes this type of exploitation; but what the revolutionary means by this word is that the present regime is a human fact. As such, it has to be rejected. This rejection cuts off the will of the oppressor, in his turn, from the future toward which he was hoping to thrust himself alone: another future is substituted, that of revolution. The struggle is not one of words and ideologies; it is real and concrete, if it is this future which triumphs, and not the former, then it is the oppressed who is realized as a positive and open freedom and the oppressor who becomes an obstacle and a thing.

There are thus two ways of surpassing the given: it is something quite different from taking a trip or escaping from prison. In these two cases the given is present in its surpassing; but in one case it is present insofar as it is accepted, in the other insofar as rejected, and that makes a radical difference. Hegel has confused these two movements with the ambiguous term "aufheben"; and the whole structure of an optimism which denies failure and death rests on this ambiguity; that is what allows one to regard the future of the world as a continuous and harmonious development; this confusion is the source and also the consequence; it is a perfect epitome of that idealistic and verbose flabbiness with which Marx charged Hegel and to which he opposed a realistic toughness. Revolt is not integrated into the harmonious development of the world; it does not wish to be integrated but rather to explode at the heart of the world and to break its continuity. It is no accident if Marx defined the attitude of the proletariat not positively but negatively: he does not show it as affirming itself or as seeking to realize a classless society, but rather as first attempting to put an end to itself as a class. And it is precisely because it has no other issue than a negative one that this situation must be eliminated.

All men are interested in this elimination, the oppressor as well as the oppressed, as Marx himself has said, for each one needs to have all men free. There are cases where the slave does not know his servitude and where it is necessary to bring the seed of his liberation to him from the outside: his submission is not enough to justify the tyranny which is imposed upon him. The slave is submissive when one has succeeded in mystifying him in such a way that his situation does not seem to him to be imposed by men, but to be immediately given by nature, by the gods, by the powers against whom revolt has no meaning; thus, he does not accept his condition through a resignation of his freedom since he can not even dream of any other; and in his relationships with his friends, for example, he can live as a free and moral man within this world where his ignorance has enclosed him. The conservative will argue from this that this peace should not be disturbed; it is not necessary to give education to the people or comfort to the natives of the colonies; the "ringleaders" should be suppressed; that is the meaning of an old story of Maurras: there is no need to awaken the sleeper, for that would be to awaken him to unhappiness. Certainly it is not a question of throwing men in spite of themselves, under the pretext of liberation, into a new world, one which they have not chosen, on which they have no grip. The proponents of slavery in the Carolinas had a good case when they showed the conquerors old negro slaves who were bewildered by a freedom which they didn't know what to do with and who cried for their former masters; these false liberations – though in a certain sense they are inevitable – overwhelm those who are their victims as if they were a new blow of blind fate. What must be done is to furnish the ignorant slave with the means of transcending his situation by means of revolt, to put an end to his ignorance. We know that the problem of the nineteenth-century socialists was precisely to develop a class consciousness in the proletariat; we see in the life of Flora Tristan, for example, how thankless such a task was: what she wanted for the workers had first to be wanted without them. "But what right does one have to want something for others?" asks the conservative, who meanwhile regards the workingman or the native as "a grown-up child" and who does not hesitate to dispose of the child's will. Indeed, there is nothing more arbitrary than intervening as a stranger in a destiny which is not ours: one of the shocking things about charity – in the civic sense of the word – is that it is practised from the outside, according to the caprice of the one who distributes it and who is detached from the object. But the cause of freedom is not that of others more than it is mine: it is universally human. If I want the slave to become conscious of his servitude, it is both in order not to be a tyrant myself – for any abstention is complicity, and complicity in this case is tyranny – and in order that new possibilities might be opened to the liberated slave and through him to all men. To want existence, to want to disclose the world, and to want men to be free are one and the same will.

Moreover, the oppressor is lying if he claims that the oppressed positively wants oppression; he merely abstains from not wanting it because he is unaware of even the possibility of rejection. All that an external action can propose is to put the oppressed in the presence of his freedom: then he will decide positively and freely. The fact is that he decides against oppression, and it is then that the movement of emancipation really begins. For if it is true that the cause of freedom is the cause of each one, it is also true that the urgency of liberation is not the same for all; Marx has rightly said that it is only to the oppressed that it appears as immediately necessary. As for us, we do not believe in a literal necessity but in a moral exigency; the oppressed can fulfill his freedom as a man only in revolt, since the essential characteristic of the situation against which he is rebelling is precisely its prohibiting him from any positive development; it is only in social and political struggle that his transcendence passes beyond to the infinite. And certainly the proletarian is no more naturally a moral man than another; he can flee from his freedom, dissipate it, vegetate without desire, and give himself up to an inhuman myth; and the trick of "enlightened" capitalism is to make him forget about his concern with genuine justification, offering him, when he leaves the factory where a mechanical job absorbs his transcendence, diversions in which this transcendence ends by petering out: there you have the politics of the American employing class which catches the worker in the trap of sports, "gadgets," autos, and frigidaires. On the whole, however, he has fewer temptations of betrayal than the members of the privileged classes because the satisfying of his passions, the taste for adventure, and the satisfactions of social seriousness are denied him. And in particular, it is also possible for the bourgeois and the intellectual to use their freedom positively at the same time as they can cooperate in the struggle against oppression: their future is not barred. That is what Ponge, for example, suggests when he writes that he is producing "post-revolutionary" literature. The writer, as well as the scientist and the technician, has the possibility of realizing, before the revolution is accomplished, this re-creation of the world which should be the task of every man if freedom were no longer enchained anywhere. Whether or not it is desirable to anticipate the future, whether men have to give up the positive use of their freedom as long as the liberation of all has not yet been achieved, or whether, on the contrary, any human fulfillment serves the cause of man, is a point about which revolutionary politics itself is still hesitating. Even in the Soviet Union itself the relation between the building of the future and the present struggle seems to be defined in very different ways according to the moment and the circumstances. It is also a matter wherein each individual has to invent his solution freely. In any case, we can assert that the oppressed is more totally engaged in the struggle than those who, though at one with him in rejecting his servitude, do not experience it; but also that, on the other hand, every man is affected by this struggle in so essential a way that he can not fulfill himself morally without taking part in it.

The problem is complicated in practice by the fact that today oppression has more than one aspect: the Arabian fellah is oppressed by both the sheiks and the French and English administration; which of the two enemies is to be combated? The interests of the French proletariat are not the same as those of the natives in the colonies: which are to be served? But here the question is political before being moral: we must end by abolishing all suppression; each one must carry on his struggle in connection with that of the other and by integrating it into the general pattern. What order should be followed? What tactics should be adopted? It is a matter of opportunity and efficiency. For each one it also depends upon his individual situation. It is possible that he may be led to sacrifice temporarily a cause whose success is subordinate to that of a cause whose defense is more urgent; on the other hand, it is possible that one may judge it necessary to maintain the tension of revolt against a situation to which one does not wish to consent at any price: thus, during the war, when Negro leaders in America were asked to drop their own claims for the sake of the general interest, Richard Wright refused; he thought that even in time of war his cause had to be defended. In any case, morality requires that the combatant be not blinded by the goal which he sets up for himself to the point of falling into the fanaticism of seriousness or passion. The cause which he serves must not lock itself up and thus create a new element of separation: through his own struggle he must seek to serve the universal cause of freedom.

At once the oppressor raises an objection: under the pretext of freedom, he says, there you go oppressing me in turn; you deprive me of *my* freedom. It is the argument which the Southern slaveholders opposed to the abolitionists, and we know that the Yankees were so imbued with the principles of an abstract democracy that they did not grant that they had the right to deny the Southern planters the freedom to own slaves; the Civil War broke out with a completely formal pretext. We smile at such scruples; yet today America still recognizes more or less implicitly that Southern whites have the freedom to lynch negroes. And it is the same sophism which is innocently displayed in the newspapers of the P.R.L. (Parti Republicain de la Liberte) and, more or less subtly, in all conservative organs. When a party promises the directing classes that it will defend their freedom, it means quite plainly that it demands that they have the freedom of exploiting the working class. A claim of this kind does not outrage us in the name of abstract justice; but a contradiction is dishonestly concealed there. For a freedom wills itself genuinely only by willing itself as an indefinite movement through the freedom of others; as soon as it withdraws into itself, it denies itself on behalf of some object which it prefers to itself: we know well enough what sort of freedom the P.R.L. demands: it is property, the feeling of possession, capital, comfort, moral security. We have to respect freedom only when it is intended for freedom, not when it strays, flees itself, and resigns itself. A freedom which is interested only in denying freedom must be denied. And it is not true that the recognition of the freedom of others limits my own freedom: to be free is not to have the power to do anything you like; it is to be able to surpass the given toward an open future; the existence of others as a freedom defines my situation and is even the condition of my own freedom. I am oppressed if I am thrown into prison, but not if I am kept from throwing my neighbor into prison.

Indeed, the oppressor himself is conscious of this sophism; he hardly dares to have recourse to it; rather than make an unvarnished demand for freedom to oppress he is more apt to present himself as the defender of certain values. It is not in his own name that he is fighting, but rather in the name of civilization, of institutions, of monuments, and of virtues which realize objectively the situation which he intends to maintain; he declares that all these things are beautiful and good in themselves; he defends a past which has assumed the icy dignity of being against an uncertain future whose values have not yet been won; this is what is well expressed by the label "conservative." As some people are curators of a museum or a collection of medals, others make themselves the curators of the given world; stressing the sacrifices that are necessarily involved in all change, they side with what has been over against what has not yet been.

It is quite certain that the surpassing of the past toward the future always demands sacrifices; to claim that in destroying an old quarter in order to build new houses on its ruins one is preserving it dialectically is a play on words; no dialectic can restore the old port of Marseilles; the past as something not surpassed, in its flesh and blood presence, has completely vanished. All that a stubborn optimism can claim is that the past does not concern us in this particular and fixed form and that we have sacrificed nothing in sacrificing it; thus, many revolutionaries consider it healthy to refuse any attachment to the past and to profess to scorn monuments and traditions. A left-wing journalist who was fuming impatiently in a street of Pompeii said, "What are we doing here? We're wasting our time." This attitude is self-confirming; let us turn away from the past, and there no longer remains any trace of it in the present, or for the future; the people of the Middle Ages had so well forgotten antiquity that there was no longer anyone who even had a desire to know something about it. One can live without Greek, without Latin, without cathedrals, and without history. Yes, but there are many other things that one can live without; the tendency of man is not to reduce himself but to increase his power. To abandon the past to the night of facticity is a way of depopulating the world. I would distrust a humanism which was too indifferent to the efforts of the men of former times; if the disclosure of being achieved by our ancestors does not at all move us, why be so interested in that which is taking place today; why wish so ardently for future realizations? To assert the reign of the human is to acknowledge man in the past as well as in the future. The Humanists of the Renaissance are an example of the help to be derived by a movement of liberation from being rooted in the past; no doubt the study of Greek and Latin does not have this living force in every age; but in any case, the fact of having a past is part of the human condition; if the world behind us were bare, we would hardly be able to see anything before us but a gloomy desert. We must try, through our living projects, to turn to our own account that freedom which was undertaken in the past and to integrate it into the present world.

But on the other hand, we know that if the past concerns us, it does so not as a brute fact, but insofar as it has human signification; if this signification can be recognized only by a project which refuses the legacy of the past, then this legacy must be refused; it would be absurd to uphold against man a datum which is precious only insofar as the freedom of man is expressed in it. There is one country where the cult of the past is erected into a system more than anywhere else: it is the Portugal of today; but it is at the cost of a deliberate contempt for man. Salazar has had brand-new castles built, at great expense, on all the hills where there were ruins standing, and at Obidos he had no hesitation in appropriating for this restoration the funds that were to go to the maternity hospital, which, as a result, had to be closed; on the outskirts of Coimbre where a children's community was to be set up, he spent so much money having the different types of old Portuguese houses reproduced on a reduced scale that barely four children could be lodged in this monstrous village. Dances, songs, local festivals, and the wearing of old regional costumes are encouraged everywhere: they never open a school. Here we see, in its extreme form, the absurdity of a choice which prefers the Thing to Man from whom alone the Thing can receive its value. We may be moved by dances, songs, and regional costumes because these inventions represent the only free accomplishment which was allowed the peasants amidst the hard conditions under which they formerly lived; by means of these creations they tore themselves away from their servile work, transcended their situation, and asserted themselves as men before the beasts of burden. Wherever these festivals still exist spontaneously, where they have retained this character, they have their meaning and their value. But when they are ceremoniously reproduced for the edification of indifferent tourists, they are no more than a boring documentary, even an odious mystification. It is a sophism to want to maintain by coercion things which derive their worth from the fact that men attempted through them to escape from coercion. In like manner, all those who oppose old lace, rugs, peasant coifs, picturesque houses, regional costumes, hand-made cloth, old language, etcetera, to social evolution know very well that they are dishonest: they themselves do not much value the present reality of these things, and most of the time their lives clearly show it. To be sure, they treat those who do not recognize the unconditional value of an Alencon point as ignoramuses; but at heart they know that these objects are less precious in themselves than as the manifestation of the civilization which they represent. They are crying up the patience and the submission of industrious hands which were one with their needle as much as they are the lace. We also know that the Nazis made very handsome bindings and lampshades out of human skin.

Thus, oppression can in no way justify itself in the name of the content which it is defending and which it dishonestly sets up as an idol. Bound up with the subjectivity which established it, this content requires its own surpassing. One does not love the past in its living truth if he insists on preserving its hardened and mummified forms. The past is an appeal; it is an appeal toward the future which sometimes can save it only by destroying it. Even though this destruction may be a sacrifice, it would be a lie to deny it: since man wants there to be being, he can not renounce any form of being without regret. But a genuine ethics does not teach us either to sacrifice it or deny it: we must assume it.

The oppressor does not merely try to justify himself as a conserver. Often he tries to invoke future realizations; he speaks in the name of the future. Capitalism sets itself up as the regime which is most favorable to production; the colonist is the only one capable of exploiting the wealth which the native would leave fallow. Oppression tries to defend itself by its utility. But we have seen that it is one of the lies of the serious mind to attempt to give the word "useful" an absolute meaning; nothing is useful if it is not useful to man; nothing is useful to man if the latter is not in a position to define his own ends and values, if he is not free. Doubtless an oppressive regime can achieve constructions which will serve man: they will serve him only from the day that he is free to use them;

as long as the reign of the oppressor lasts, none of the benefits of oppression is a real benefit. Neither in the past nor in the future can one prefer a thing to man, who alone can establish the reason for all things.

Finally, the oppressor has a good case for showing that respect for freedom is never without difficulty, and perhaps he may even assert that one can never respect all freedoms at the same time. But that simply means that man must accept the tension of the struggle, that his liberation must actively seek to perpetuate itself, without aiming at an impossible state of equilibrium and rest; this does not mean that he ought to prefer the sleep of slavery to this incessant conquest. Whatever the problems raised for him, the setbacks that he will have to assume, and the difficulties with which he will have to struggle, he must reject oppression at any cost.

The Antinomies of Action

As we have seen, if the oppressor were aware of the demands of his own freedom, he himself should have to denounce oppression. But he is dishonest; in the name of the serious or of his passions, of his will for power or of his appetites, he refuses to give up his privileges. In order for a liberating action to be a thoroughly moral action, it would have to be achieved through a conversion of the oppressors: there would then be a reconciliation of all freedoms. But no one any longer dares to abandon himself today to these utopian reveries. We know only too well that we can not count upon a collective conversion. However, by virtue of the fact that the oppressors refuse to co-operate in the affirmation of freedom, they embody, in the eyes of all men of good will, the absurdity of facticity; by calling for the triumph of freedom over facticity, ethics also demands that they be suppressed; and since their subjectivity, by definition, escapes our control, it will be possible to act only on their objective presence; others will here have to be treated like things, with violence; the sad fact of the separation of men will thereby be confirmed. Thus, here is the oppressor oppressed in turn; and the men who do violence to him in their turn become masters, tyrants, and executioners: in revolting, the oppressed are metamorphosed into a blind force, a brutal fatality; the evil which divides the world is carried out in their own hearts. And doubtless it is not a question of backing out of these consequences, for the ill-will of the oppressor imposes upon each one the alternative of being the enemy of the oppressed if he is not that of their tyrant; evidently, it is necessary to choose to sacrifice the one who is an enemy of man; but the fact is that one finds himself forced to treat certain men as things in order to win the freedom of all.

A freedom which is occupied in denying freedom is itself so outrageous that the outrageousness of the violence which one practices against it is almost cancelled out: hatred, indignation, and anger (which even the Marxist cultivates, despite the cold impartiality of the doctrine) wipe out all scruples. But the oppressor would not be so strong if he did not have accomplices among the oppressed themselves; mystification is one of the forms of oppression; ignorance is a situation in which man may be enclosed as narrowly as in a prison; as we have already said, every individual may practice his freedom inside his world, but not everyone has the means of rejecting, even by doubt, the values, taboos, and prescriptions by which he is surrounded; doubtless, respectful minds take the object of their respect for their own; in this sense they are *responsible* for it, as they are responsible for their presence in the world: but they are not *guilty* if their adhesion is not a resignation of their freedom. When a young sixteen-year old Nazi died crying, "Heil Hitler!" he was not guilty, and it was not he whom we hated but his masters. The desirable thing would be to re-educate this misled youth; it would be necessary to expose the mystification and to put the men who are its victims in the presence of their freedom. But the urgency of the struggle forbids this slow labor. We are obliged to destroy not only the oppressor but also those who serve him, whether they do so out of ignorance or out of constraint.

As we have also seen, the situation of the world is so complex that one can not fight everywhere at the same time and for everyone. In order to win an urgent victory, one has to give up the idea, at least temporarily, of serving certain valid causes; one may even be brought to the point of fighting against them. Thus, during the course of the last war, no Anti-fascist could have wanted the revolts of the natives in the British Empire to be successful; on the contrary, these revolts were supported by the Fascist regimes; and yet, we can not blame those who, considering their emancipation to be the more urgent action, took advantage of the situation to obtain it. Thus, it is possible, and often it even happens, that one finds himself obliged to oppress and kill men who are pursuing goals whose validity one acknowledges himself.

But that is not the worst thing to be said for violence. It not only forces us to sacrifice the men who are in our way, but also those who are fighting on our side, and even ourselves. Since we can conquer our enemies only by acting upon their facticity, by reducing them to things, we have to make ourselves things; in this struggle in which wills are forced to confront each other through their bodies, the bodies of our allies, like those of our opponents are exposed to the same brutal hazard: they will be wounded, killed, or starved. Every war, every revolution, demands the sacrifice of a generation, of a collectivity, by those who undertake it. And even outside of periods of crisis when blood flows, the permanent possibility of violence can constitute between nations and classes a state of veiled warfare in which individuals are sacrificed in a permanent way.

Thus one finds himself in the presence of the paradox that no action can be generated for man without its being immediately generated against men. This obvious truth, which is universally known, is, however, so bitter that the first concern of a doctrine of action is ordinarily to mask this element of failure that is involved in any undertaking. The parties of oppression beg the question; they deny the value of what they sacrifice in such a way that they find that they are *sacrificing* nothing. Passing dishonestly from the serious to nihilism, they set up both the unconditioned value of their end and the insignificance of the men whom they are using as instruments. High as it may be, the number of victims is always measurable; and each one taken one by one is never anything but an individual: yet, through time and space, the triumph of the cause embraces the infinite, it interests the whole collectivity. In order to deny the outrage it is enough to deny the importance of the individual, even though it be at the cost of this collectivity: *it* is everything, *he* is only a zero.

In one sense the individual, as a matter of fact, is not very much, and we can understand the misanthrope who in 1939 declared: "After all, when you look at people one by one, it doesn't seem so awful a thing to make war upon them." Reduced to pure facticity, congealed in his immanence, cut off from his future, deprived of his transcendence and of the world which that transcendence discloses, a man no longer appears as anything more than a thing among things which can be subtracted from the collectivity of other things without its leaving upon the earth any trace of its absence. Multiply this paltry existence by thousands of copies and its insignificance remains; mathematics also teaches us that zero multiplied by any finite number remains zero. It is even possible that the wretchedness of each element is only further affirmed by this futile expansion. Horror is sometimes self-destructive before the photographs of the charnel-houses of Buchenwald and Dachau and of the ditches strewn with bones; it takes on the aspect of indifference; that decomposed, that animal flesh seems so essentially doomed to decay that one can no longer even regret that it has fulfilled its destiny; it is when a man is alive that his death appears to be an outrage, but a corpse has the stupid tranquillity of trees and stones: those who have done it say that it is easy to walk on a corpse and still easier to walk over a pile of corpses; and it is the same reason that accounts for the callousness described by those deportees who escaped death: through sickness, pain, hunger, and death, they no longer saw their comrades and themselves as anything more than an animal horde whose life or desires were no longer justified by anything, whose very revolts were only the agitations of animals. In order to remain capable of perceiving man through these humiliated bodies one had to be sustained by political faith, intellectual pride, or Christian charity. That is why the Nazis were so systematically relentless in casting into abjection the men they wanted to destroy: the disgust which the victims felt in regard to themselves stifled the voice of revolt and justified the executioners in their own eyes. All oppressive regimes become stronger through the degradation of the oppressed. In Algeria I have seen any number of colonists appease their conscience by the contempt in which they held the Arabs who were crushed with misery: the more miserable the latter were, the more contemptible they seemed, so much so that there was never any room for remorse. And the truth is that certain tribes in the south were so ravaged by disease and famine that one could no longer feel either rebellious or hopeful regarding them; rather, one wished for the death of those unhappy creatures who have been reduced to so elemental an animality that even the maternal instinct has been suppressed in them. Yet, with all this sordid resignation, there were children who played and laughed; and their smile exposed the lie of their oppressors: it was an appeal and a promise; it projected a future before the child, a man's future. If, in all oppressed countries, a child's face is so moving, it is not that the child is more moving or that he has more of a right to happiness than the others: it is that he is the living affirmation of human transcendence: he is on the watch, he is an eager hand held out to the world, he is a hope, a project. The trick of tyrants is to enclose a man in the immanence of his facticity and to try to forget that man is always, as Heidegger puts it, "infinitely more than what he would be if he were reduced to being what he is;" man is a being of the distances, a movement toward the future, a project. The tyrant asserts himself as a transcendence; he considers others as pure immanences: he thus arrogates to himself the right to treat them like cattle. We see the sophism on which his conduct is based: of the ambiguous condition which is that of all men, he retains for himself the only aspect of a transcendence which is capable of justifying itself; for the others, the contingent and unjustified aspect of immanence.

But if that kind of contempt for man is convenient, it is also dangerous; the feeling of abjection can confirm men in a hopeless resignation but can not incite them to the struggle and sacrifice which is consented to with their life; this was seen in the time of the Roman decadence when men lost their zest for life and the readiness to risk it. In any case, the tyrant himself does not openly set up this contempt as a universal principle: it is the Jew, the negro, or the native whom he encloses in his immanence; with his subordinates and his soldiers he uses different language. For it is quite clear that if the individual is a pure zero, the sum of those zeros which make up the collectivity is also a zero: no undertaking has any importance, no defeat as well as no victory. In order to appeal to the devotion of his troops, the chief or the authoritarian party will utilize a truth which is the opposite of the one which sanctions their brutal oppression: namely, that the value of the individual is asserted only in his surpassing. This is one of the aspects of the doctrine of Hegel which the dictatorial regimes readily make use of. And it is a point at which fascist ideology and Marxist ideology converge. A doctrine which aims at the liberation of man evidently can not rest on a contempt for the individual; but it can propose to him no other salvation than his subordination to the collectivity. The finite is nothing if it is not its transition to the infinite; the death of an individual is not a failure if it is integrated into a project which surpasses the limits of life, the substance of this life being outside of the individual himself, in the class, in the socialist State; if the individual is taught to consent to his sacrifice, the latter is abolished as such, and the soldier who has renounced himself in favor of his cause will die joyfully; in fact, that is how the young Hitlerians died.

We know how many edifying speeches this philosophy has inspired: it is by losing oneself that one finds himself, by dying that one fulfills his life, by accepting servitude that one realizes his freedom; all leaders of men preach in this vein. And if there are any who refuse to heed this language, they are wrong, they are cowards: as such, they are worthless, they aren't worth anyone's bothering with them. The brave man dies gaily, of his own free will; the one who rejects death deserves only to die. There you have the problem elegantly resolved.

But one may ask whether this convenient solution is not self-contesting. In Hegel the individual is only an abstract moment in the History of absolute Mind. This is explained by the first intuition of the system which, identifying the real and the rational, empties the human world of its sensible thickness; if the truth of the here and now is only Space and Time, if the truth of one's cause is its passage into the other, then the attachment to the individual substance of life is evidently an error, an inadequate attitude. The essential moment of Hegelian ethics is the moment when consciousnesses recognize one another; in this operation the other is recognized as identical with me, which means that in myself it is the universal truth of my self which alone is recognized; so individuality is denied, and it can no longer reappear except on the natural and contingent plane; moral salvation will lie in my surpassing toward that other who is equal to myself and who in turn will surpass himself toward another. Hegel himself recognizes that if this passage continued indefinitely, Totality would never be achieved, the real would peter out in the same measure: one can not, without absurdity, indefinitely sacrifice each generation to the following one; human history would then be only an endless succession of negations which would never return to the positive; all action would be destruction and life would be a vain flight. We must admit that there will be a recovery of the real and that all sacrifices will find their positive form within the absolute Mind. But this does not work without some difficulty. The Mind is a subject; but *who* is a subject? After Descartes how can we ignore the fact that subjectivity radically signifies separation? And if it is admitted, at the cost of a contradiction, that *the* subject will be *the* men of the future reconciled, it must be clearly recognized that the men of today who turn out to have been the *substance* of the real, and not *subjects,* remain excluded forever from this reconciliation. Furthermore, even Hegel retreats from the idea of this motionless future; since Mind is restlessness, the dialectic of struggle and conciliation can never be stopped: the future which it envisages is not the perpetual peace of Kant but an indefinite state of war. It declares that this war will no longer appear as a temporary evil in which each individual makes a gift of himself to the State; but it is precisely at this point that there is a bit of sleight-of-hand: for *why* would he agree to this gift since the State can not be the achieving of the real Totality recovering itself? The whole system seems like a huge mystification, since it subordinates all its moments to an end term whose coming it dares not set up; the individual renounces himself; but no reality in favor of which he can renounce himself is ever affirmed or recovered. Through all this learned dialectic we finally come back to the sophism which we exposed: if the individual is nothing, society can not be something. Take his substance away from him, and the State has no more substance; if he has nothing to sacrifice, there is nothing before him to sacrifice to. Hegelian fullness immediately passes into the nothingness of absence. And the very grandeur of that failure makes this truth shine forth: only the subject can justify his own existence; no external subject, no object, can bring him salvation from the outside. He can not be regarded as a nothing, since the consciousness of all things is within him.

Thus, nihilistic pessimism and rationalistic optimism fail in their effort to juggle away the bitter truth of sacrifice: they also eliminate all reasons for wanting it. Someone told a young invalid who wept because she had to leave her home, her occupations, and her whole past life, "Get cured. The rest has no importance." "But if nothing has any importance," she answered, "what good is it to get cured?" She was right. In order for this world to have any importance, in order for our undertaking to have a meaning and to be worthy of sacrifices, we must affirm the concrete and particular thickness of this world and the individual reality of our projects and ourselves. This is what democratic societies understand; they strive to confirm citizens in the feeling of their individual value; the whole ceremonious apparatus of baptism, marriage, and burial is the collectivity's homage to the individual; and the rites of justice seek to manifest society's respect for each of its members considered in his particularity. After or during a period of violence when men are treated like objects, one is astonished, even irritated, at seeing human life rediscover, in certain cases, a sacred character. Why those hesitations of the courts, those long drawn-out trials, since men died by the million, like animals, since the very ones being judged coldly massacred them? The reason is that once the period of crisis, in which the democracies themselves, whether they liked it or not, had to resort to blind violence, has passed, they aim to re-establish the individual within his rights; more than ever they must restore to their members the sense of their dignity, the sense of the dignity of each man, taken one by one; the soldier must become a citizen again so that the city may continue to subsist as such, may continue to deserve one's dedicating oneself to it.

But if the individual is set up as a unique and irreducible value, the word sacrifice regains all its meaning; what a man loses in renouncing his plans, his future, and his life no longer appears as a negligible thing. Even if he decides that in order to justify his life he must consent to limiting its course, even if he accepts dying, there is a wrench at the heart of this acceptance, for freedom demands both that it recover itself as an absolute and that it prolong its movement indefinitely: it is through this indefinite movement that it desires to come back to itself and to confirm itself; now, death puts an end to his drive; the hero can transcend death toward a future fulfillment, but he will not be present in that future; this must be understood if one wishes to restore to heroism its true worth: it is neither natural nor easy; the hero may overcome his regret and carry out his sacrifice; the latter is none the less an absolute renunciation. The death of those to whom we are attached by particular ties will also be consented to as an individual and irreducible misfortune. A collectivist conception of man does not concede a valid existence to such sentiments as love, tenderness, and friendship; the abstract identity of individuals merely authorizes a comradeship between them by means of which each one is likened to each of the others. In marching, in choral singing, in common work and struggle, all the others appear as the same; nobody ever dies. On the contrary, if individuals recognize themselves in their differences, individual relations are established among them, and each one becomes irreplaceable for a few others. And violence does not merely provoke in the world the wrench of the sacrifice to which one has consented; it is also undergone in revolt and refusal. Even the one who desires a victory and who knows that it has to be paid for will wonder: why with *my* blood rather than with another's? Why is it my son who is dead? And we have seen that every struggle obliges us to sacrifice people whom our victory does not concern, people who, in all honesty, reject it as a cataclysm: these people will die in astonishment, anger or despair. Undergone as a misfortune, violence appears as a crime to the one who practices it. That is why Saint-Just, who believed in the individual and who knew that all authority is violence, said with somber lucidity, "No one governs innocently."

We may well assume that not all those who govern have the courage to make such a confession; and furthermore it might be dangerous for them to make it too loudly. They try to mask the crime from themselves; at least they try to conceal it from the notice of those who submit to their law. If they can not totally deny it, they attempt to justify it. The most radical justification would be to demonstrate that it is necessary: it then ceases to be a crime, it becomes fatality. Even if an end is posited as necessary, the contingency of the means renders the chief's decisions arbitrary, and each individual suffering appears as unjustified: why this bloody revolution instead of slow reforms? And who will dare to designate the victim who is anonymously demanded by the general plan? On the contrary, if only one way shows itself to be possible, if the unrolling of history is fatal, there is no longer any place for the anguish of choice, or for regret, or for outrage; revolt can no longer surge up in any heart. This is what makes historical materialism so reassuring a doctrine; the troublesome idea of a subjective caprice or an objective chance is thereby eliminated. The thought and the voice of the directors merely reflect the fatal exigencies of History. But in order that this faith be living and efficacious, it is necessary that no reflection mediatize the subjectivity of the chiefs and make it appear as such; if the chief considers that he does not simply reflect the given situation but that he is interpreting it, he becomes a prey to anguish: who am I to believe in myself? And if the soldier's eyes open, he too asks: who is he to command me? Instead of a prophet, he sees nothing more than a tyrant. That is why every authoritarian party regards thought as a danger and reflection as a crime; it is by means of thought that crime appears as such in the world. This is one of the meanings of Koestler's *Darkness at Noon*. Roubatchov easily slips into confession because he feels that hesitation and doubt are the most radical, the most unpardonable of faults; they undermine the world of objectivity much more than does an act of capricious disobedience. Yet, however cruel the yoke may be, in spite of the purges, murders, and deportations, every regime has opponents: there are reflection, doubt, and contestation. And even if the opponent is in the wrong, his error brings to light a truth, namely, that there is a place in this world for error and subjectivity; whether he is right or wrong, he triumphs; he shows that the men who are in power may also be mistaken. And furthermore, the latter know it; they know that they hesitate and that their decisions are risky. The doctrine of necessity is much more a weapon than a faith; and if they use it, they do so because they know well enough that the soldier may act otherwise than he does, otherwise than the way they want him to, that he may disobey; they know well enough that he is free and that they are fettering his freedom. It is the first sacrifice that they impose upon him: in order to achieve the liberation of men he has to give up his own freedom, even his freedom of thought. In order to mask the violence, what they do is to have recourse to a new violence which even invades his mind.

Very well, replies the partisan who is sure of his aims, but this violence is useful. And the justification which he here invokes is that which, in the most general way, inspires and legitimizes all action. From conservatives to revolutionaries, through idealistic and moral vocabularies or realistic and positive ones, the outrageousness of violence is excused in the name of utility. It does not much matter that the action is not fatally commanded by anterior events as long as it is called for by the proposed end; this end sets up the means which are subordinated to it; and thanks to this subordination, one can perhaps not avoid sacrifice but one can legitimize it: this is what is important to the man of action; like Saint-Just, he accepts the loss of his innocence. It is the arbitrariness of the crime that is repugnant to him more than the crime itself. If the sacrifices which have been assented to find their rational place within the enterprise, one escapes from the anguish of decision and from remorse. But one has to win out; defeat would change the murders and destruction into unjustified outrage, since they would have been carried out in vain; but victory gives meaning and utility to all the misfortunes which have helped bring it about.

Such a position would be solid and satisfactory if the word *useful* had an absolute meaning in itself; as we have seen, the characteristic of the spirit of seriousness is precisely to confer a meaning upon it by raising the Thing or the Cause to the dignity of an unconditioned end. The only problem then raised is a technical problem; the means will be chosen according to their effectiveness, their speed, and their economy; it is simply a question of measuring the relationships of the factors of time, cost, and probability of success. Furthermore, in war-time discipline spares the subordinates the problems of such calculations; they concern only the staff. The soldier does not call into question either the aim or the means of attaining it: he obeys without any discussion. However, what distinguishes war and politics from all other techniques is that the material that is employed is a human material. Now human efforts and lives can no more be treated as blind instruments than human work can be treated as simple merchandise; at the same time as he is a means for attaining an end, man is himself an end. The word *useful* requires a complement, and there can be only one: man himself. And the most disciplined soldier would mutiny if skillful propaganda did not persuade him that he is dedicating himself to the cause of man: to his cause.

But is the cause of Man that of each man? That is what utilitarian ethics has been striving to demonstrate since Hegel; if one wishes to give the word *useful* a universal and absolute meaning, it is always a question of reabsorbing each man into the bosom of mankind; it is said that despite the weaknesses of the flesh and that particular fear which each one experiences in the face of his particular death, the real interest of each one is mingled with the general interest. And it is true that each is bound to all; but that is precisely the ambiguity of his condition: in his surpassing toward others, each one exists absolutely as for himself; each is interested in the liberation of all, but as a separate existence engaged in his own projects. So much so that the terms "useful to Man," "useful to this man," do not overlap. Universal, absolute man exists nowhere. From this angle, we again come upon the same antinomy: the only justification of sacrifice is its utility; but the useful is what serves Man. Thus, in order to serve some men we must do disservice to others. By what principle are we to choose between them?

It must again be called to mind that the supreme end at which man must aim is his freedom, which alone is capable of establishing the value of every end; thus, comfort, happiness, all relative goods which human projects define, will be subordinated to this absolute condition of realization. The freedom of a single man must count more than a cotton or rubber harvest; although this principle is not respected in fact, it is usually recognized theoretically. But what makes the problem so difficult is that it is a matter of choosing between the negation of one freedom or another: every war supposes a discipline, every revolution a dictatorship, every political move a certain amount of lying; action implies all forms of enslaving, from murder to mystification. Is it therefore absurd in every case? Or, in spite of everything, are we able to find, within the very outrage that it implies, reasons for wanting one thing rather than another?

One generally takes numerical considerations into account by a strange compromise which clearly shows that every action treats men both as a means and as an end, as an external object and as an inwardness; it is better to save the lives of ten men than of only one. Thus, one treats man as an end, for to set up quantity as a value is to set up the positive value of each unit; but it is setting it up as a quantifiable value, thus, as an externality. I have known a Kantian rationalist who passionately maintained that it is as immoral to choose the death of a single man as to let ten thousand die; he was right in the sense that in each murder the outrage is total; ten thousand dead – there are never ten thousand copies of a single death; no multiplication is relevant to subjectivity. But he forgot that for the one who had the decision to make men are given, nevertheless, as objects that can be counted; it is therefore logical, though this logic implies an outrageous absurdity, to prefer the salvation of the greater number. Moreover, this position of the problem is rather abstract, for one rarely bases a choice on pure quantity. Those men among whom one hesitates have functions in society. The general who is sparing of the lives of his soldiers saves them as human material that it is useful to save for tomorrow's battles or for the reconstruction of the country; and he sometimes condemns to death thousands of civilians whose fate he is not concerned with in order to spare the lives of a hundred soldiers or ten specialists. An extreme case is the one David Rousset describes in *The Days of Our Death:* the S.S. obliged the responsible members of the concentration camps to designate which prisoners were to go to the gas chambers. The politicians agreed to assume this responsibility because they thought that they had a valid principle of selection: they protected the politicians of their party because the lives of these men who were devoted to a cause which they thought was just seemed to them to be the most useful to preserve. We know that the communists have been widely accused of this partiality; however, since one could in no way escape the atrocity of these massacres, the only thing to do was to try, as far as possible, to rationalize it.

It seems as if we have hardly advanced, for we come back, in the end, to the statement that what appears as useful is to sacrifice the less useful men to the more useful. But even this shift from useful to useful will enlighten us: the complement of the word *useful* is the word *man,* but it is also the word *future.* It is man insofar as he is, according to the formula of Ponge, "the future of man." Indeed, cut off from his transcendence, reduced to the facticity of his presence, an individual is nothing; it is by his project that he fulfills himself, by the end at which he aims that he justifies himself; thus, this justification is always to come. Only the future can take the present for its own and keep it alive by surpassing it. A choice will become possible in the light of the future, which is the meaning of tomorrow because the present appears as the facticity which must be transcended toward freedom. No action is conceivable without this sovereign affirmation of the future. But we still have to agree upon what underlies this word.

The Present and the Future

The word *future* has two meanings corresponding to the two aspects of the ambiguous condition of man which is lack of being and which is existence; it alludes to both being and existence. When I envisage my future, I consider that movement which, prolonging my existence of today, will fulfill my present projects and will surpass them toward new ends: the future is the definite direction of a particular transcendence and it is so closely bound up with the present that it composes with it a single temporal form; this is the future which Heidegger considered as a reality which is given at each moment. But through the centuries men have dreamed of another future in which it might be granted them to retrieve themselves as beings in Glory, Happiness, or Justice; this future did not prolong the present; it came down upon the world like a cataclysm announced by signs which cut the continuity of time: by a Messiah, by meteors, by the trumpets of the Last Judgment. By transporting the kingdom of God to heaven, Christians have almost stripped it of its temporal character, although it was promised to the believer only at the end of his life. It was the anti-Christian humanism of the eighteenth century which brought the myth down to earth again. Then, through the idea of progress, an idea of the future was elaborated in which its two aspects fused: the future appeared both as the meaning of our transcendence and as the immobility of being; it is human, terrestrial, and the resting-place of things. It is in this form that it is hesitantly reflected in the systems of Hegel and of Comte. It is in this form that it is so often invoked today as a unity of the World or as a finished socialist State. In both cases the Future appears as both the infinite and as Totality, as number and as unity of conciliation; it is the abolition of the negative, it is fullness, happiness. One might surmise that any sacrifice already made might be claimed in its name. However great the quantity of men sacrificed today, the quantity that will profit by their sacrifice is infinitely greater; on the other hand, in the face of the positivity of the future, the present is only the negative which must be eliminated as such: only by dedicating itself to this positivity can the negative henceforth return to the positive. The present is the transitory existence which is made in order to be abolished: it retrieves itself only by transcending itself toward the permanence of future being; it is only as an instrument, as a means, it is only by its efficacity with regard to the coming of the future that the present is validly realized: reduced to itself it is nothing, one may dispose of it as he pleases. That is the ultimate meaning of the formula: the end justifies the means: all means are authorized by their very indifference. Thus, some serenely think that the present oppression has no importance if, through it, the World can be fulfilled as such: then, within the harmonious equilibrium of work and wealth, oppression will be wiped out by itself. Others serenely think that the present dictatorship of a party with its lies and violence has no importance if, by means of it, the socialist State is realized: arbitrariness and crime will then disappear forever from the face of the earth. And still others think more sloppily that the shilly-shallyings and the compromises have no importance since the future will turn out well and, in some way or other, will muddle along into victory. Those who project themselves toward a Future-Thing and submerge their freedom in it find the tranquillity of the serious.

However, we have seen that, despite the requirements of his system, even Hegel does not dare delude himself with the idea of a stationary future; he admits that, mind being restlessness, the struggle will never cease. Marx did not consider the coming of the socialist state as an absolute result, but as the end of a pre-history on the basis of which real history begins. However, it would be sufficient, in order for the myth of the future to be valid, for this history to be conceivable as a harmonious development where reconciled men would fulfill themselves as a pure positivity; but this dream is not permitted since man is originally a negativity. No social upheaval, no moral conversion can eliminate this lack which is in his heart; it is by making himself a lack of being that man exists, and positive existence is this lack assumed but not eliminated; we can not establish upon existence an abstract wisdom which, turning itself away from being, would aim at only the harmony itself of the existants: for it is then the absolute silence of the in-itself which would close up around this negation of negativity; without this particular movement which thrusts him toward the future man would not exist. But then one can not imagine any reconciliation of transcendences: they do not have the indifferent docility of a pure abstraction; they are concrete and concretely compete with others for being. The world which they reveal is a battle-field where there is no neutral ground and which cannot be divided up into parcels: for each individual project is asserted through the world as a whole. The fundamental ambiguity of the human condition will always open up to men the possibility of opposing choices; there will always be within them the desire to be that being of whom they have made themselves a lack, the flight from the anguish of freedom; the plane of hell, of struggle, will never be eliminated; freedom will never be given; it will always have to be won: that is what Trotsky was saying when he envisaged the future as a permanent revolution. Thus, there is a fallacy hidden in that abuse of language which all parties make use of today to justify their politics when they declare that the world is still at war. If one means by that that the struggle is not over, that the world is a prey to opposed interests which affront each other violently, he is speaking the truth; but he also means that such a situation is abnormal and calls for abnormal behavior; the politics that it involves can impugn every moral principle, since it has only a provisional form: later on we shall act in accordance with truth and justice. To the idea of present war there is opposed that of a future peace when man will again find, along with a stable situation, the possibility of a morality. But the truth is that if division and violence define war, the world has always been at war and always will be; if man is waiting for universal peace in order to establish his existence validly, he will wait indefinitely: there will never be any *other* future.

It is possible that some may challenge this assertion as being based upon debatable ontological presuppositions; it should at least be recognized that this harmonious future is only an uncertain dream and that in any case it is not ours. Our hold on the future is limited; the movement of expansion of existence requires that we strive at every moment to amplify it; but where it stops our future stops too; beyond, there is nothing more because nothing more is disclosed. From that formless night we can draw no justification of our acts, it condemns them with the same indifference; wiping out today's errors and defeats, it will also wipe out its triumphs; it can be chaos or death as well as paradise: perhaps men will one day return to barbarism, perhaps one day the earth will no longer be anything but an icy planet. In this perspective all moments are lost in the indistinctness of nothingness and being. Man ought not entrust the care of his salvation to this uncertain and foreign future: it is up to him to assure it within his own existence; this existence is conceivable, as we have said, only as an affirmation of the future, but of a human future, a finite future.

It is difficult today to safeguard this sense of finiteness. The Greek cities and the Roman republic were able to will themselves in their finiteness because the infinite which invested them was for them only darkness; they died because of this ignorance, but they also lived by it. Today, however, we are having a hard time living because we are so bent on outwitting death. We are aware that the whole world is interested in each of our undertakings and this spatial enlargement of our projects also governs their temporal dimension; by a paradoxical symmetry, whereas an individual accords great value to one day of his life, and a city to one year, the interests of the World are computed in centuries; the greater the human density that one envisages, the more the viewpoint of externality wins over that of internality, and the idea of externality carries with it that of quantity. Thus, the scales of measurement have changed; space and time have expanded about us: today it is a small matter that a million men and a century seem to us only a provisional moment; yet, the individual is not touched by this transformation, his life keeps the same rhythm, his death does not retreat before him; he extends his control of the world by instruments which enable him to devour distances and to multiply the output of his effort in time; but he is always only one. However, instead of accepting his limits, he tries to do away with them. He aspires to act upon everything and by knowing everything. Throughout the eighteenth and nineteenth centuries there developed the dream of a universal science which, manifesting the solidarity of the parts of the whole also admitted a universal power; it was a dream "dreamed by reason," as Valery puts it, but which was none the less hollow, like all dreams. For a scientist who would aspire to know everything about a phenomenon would dissolve it within the totality; and a man who would aspire to act upon the totality of the Universe would see the meaning of all action vanish. Just as the infinity spread out before my gaze contracts above my head into a blue ceiling, so my transcendence heaps up in the distance the opaque thickness of the future; but between sky and earth there is a perceptional field with its forms and colors; and it is in the interval which separates me today from an unforeseeable future that there are meanings and ends toward which to direct my acts. As soon as one introduces the presence of the finite individual into the world, a presence without which there is no world, finite forms stand out through time and space. And in reverse, though a landscape is not only a transition but a particular object, an event is not only a passage but a particular reality. If one denies with Hegel the concrete thickness of the here and now in favor of universal space-time, if one denies the separate consciousness in favor of Mind, one misses with Hegel the truth of the world.

It is no more necessary to regard History as a rational totality than to regard the Universe as such. Man, mankind, the universe, and history are, in Sartre's expression, "detotalized totalities," that is, separation does not exclude relation, nor vice-versa. Society exists only by means of the existence of particular individuals; likewise, human adventures stand out against the background of time, each finite to each, though they are all open to the infinity of the future and their individual forms thereby imply each other without destroying each other. A conception of this kind does not contradict that of a historical unintelligibility; for it is not true that the mind has to choose between the contingent absurdity of the discontinuous and the rationalistic necessity of the continuous; on the contrary, it is part of its function to make a multiplicity of coherent ensembles stand out against the unique background of the world and, inversely, to comprehend these ensembles in the perspective of an ideal unity of the world. Without raising the question of historical comprehension and causality it is enough to recognize the presence of intelligible sequences within temporal forms so that forecasts and consequently action may be possible. In fact, whatever may be the philosophy we adhere to, whether our uncertainty manifests an objective and fundamental contingency or whether it expresses our subjective ignorance in the face of a rigorous necessity, the practical attitude remains the same; we must decide upon the opportuneness of an act and attempt to measure its effectiveness without knowing all the factors that are present. Just as the scientist, in order to know a phenomenon, does not wait for the light of completed knowledge to break upon it; on the contrary, in illuminating the phenomenon, he helps establish the knowledge; in like manner, the man of action, in order to make a decision, will not wait for a perfect knowledge to prove to him the necessity of a certain choice; he must first choose and thus help fashion history. A choice of this kind is no more arbitrary than a hypothesis; it excludes neither reflection nor even method; but it is also free, and it implies risks that must be assumed as such. The movement of the mind, whether it be called thought or will, always starts up in the darkness. And at bottom it matters very little, practically speaking, whether there is a Science of history or not, since this Science can come to light only at the end of the future and since at each particular moment we must, in any case, maneuver in a state of doubt. The communists themselves admit that it is subjectively possible for them to be mistaken despite the strict dialectic of History. The latter is not revealed to them today in its finished form; they are obliged to foresee its development, and this foresight may be erroneous. Thus, from the political and tactical point of view there will be no difference between a doctrine of pure dialectical necessity and a doctrine which leaves room for contingency; the difference is of a moral order. For, in the first case one admits a retrieval of each moment in the future, and thus one does not aspire to justify it by itself; in the second case, each undertaking, involving only a finite future, must be lived in its finiteness and considered as an absolute which no unknown time will ever succeed in saving. In fact, the one who asserts the unity of history also recognizes that distinct ensembles stand out within it; and the one who emphasizes the particularity of these ensembles admits that they all project against a single horizon; just as for all there exist both individuals and a collectivity; the affirmation of the collectivity over against the individual is opposed, not on the plane of fact, but on the moral plane, to the assertion of a collectivity of individuals each existing for himself. The case is the same in what concerns time and its moments, and just as we believe that by denying each individual one by one, one eliminates the collectivity, we think that if man gives himself up to an indefinite pursuit of the future he will lose his existence without ever recovering it; he then resembles a madman who runs after his shadow. The means, it is said, will be justified by the end; but it is the means which define it, and if it is contradicted at the moment that it is set up, the whole enterprise sinks into absurdity. In this way the attitude of England in regard to Spain, Greece, and Palestine is defended with the pretext that she must take up position against the Russian menace in order to save, along with her own existence, her civilization and the values of democracy; but a democracy which defends itself only by acts of oppression equivalent to those of authoritarian regimes, is precisely denying all these values; whatever the virtues of a civilization may be, it immediately belies them if it buys them by means of injustice and tyranny. Inversely, if the justifying end is thrown ahead to the farthermost end of a mythical future, it is no longer a reflection upon the means; being nearer and clearer, the means itself becomes the goal aimed at; it blocks the horizon without, however, being deliberately wanted. The triumph of Russia is proposed as a means of liberating the international proletariat; but has it not become an absolute end for all Stalinists? The end justifies the means only if it remains present, if it is completely disclosed in the course of the present enterprise.

And as a matter of fact, if it is true that men seek in the future a guarantee of their success, a negation of their failures, it is true that they also feel the need of denying the indefinite flight of time and of holding their present between their hands. Existence must be asserted in the present if one does not want all life to be defined as an escape toward nothingness. That is the reason societies institute festivals whose role is to stop the movement of transcendence, to set up the end as an end. The hours following the liberation of Paris, for example, were an immense collective festival exalting the happy and absolute end of that particular history which was precisely the occupation of Paris. There were at the moment worried spirits who were already surpassing the present toward future difficulties; they refused to rejoice under the pretext that new problems were going to come up immediately; but this ill-humor was met with only among those who had very slight wish to see the Germans defeated. All those who had made this combat their combat, even if only by the sincerity of their hopes, also regarded the victory as an absolute victory, whatever the future might be. Nobody was so naive as not to know that unhappiness would soon find other forms; but this particular unhappiness was wiped off the earth, absolutely. That is the modern meaning of the festival, private as well as public. Existence attempts in the festival to confirm itself positively as existence. That is why, as Bataille has shown, it is characterized by destruction; the ethics of being is the ethics of saving: by storing up, one aims at the stationary plenitude of the in-itself, existence, on the contrary, is consumption; it makes itself only by destroying; the festival carries out this negative movement in order to indicate clearly its independence in relationship to the thing: one eats, drinks, lights fires, breaks things, and spends time and money; one spends them for nothing. The spending is also a matter of establishing a communication of the existants, for it is by the movement of recognition which goes from one to the other that existence is confirmed; in songs, laughter, dances, eroticism, and drunkenness one seeks both an exaltation of the moment and a complicity with other men. But the tension of existence realized as a pure negativity can not maintain itself for long; it must be immediately engaged in a new undertaking, it must dash off toward the future. The moment of detachment, the pure affirmation of the subjective present are only abstractions; the joy becomes exhausted, drunkenness subsides into fatigue, and one finds himself with his hands empty because one can never possess the present: that is what gives festivals their pathetic and deceptive character. One of art's roles is to fix this passionate assertion of existence in a more durable way: the festival is at the origin of the theatre, music, the dance, and poetry. In telling a story, in depicting it, one makes it exist in its particularity with its beginning and its end, its glory or its shame; and this is the way it actually must be lived. In the festival, in art, men express their need to feel that they exist absolutely. They must really fulfill this wish. What stops them is that as soon as they give the word "end" its double meaning of goal and fulfillment they clearly perceive this ambiguity of their condition, which is the most fundamental of all: that every living movement is a sliding toward death. But if they are willing to look it in the face they also discover that every movement toward death is life. In the past people cried out, "The king is dead, long live the king;" thus the present must die so that it may live; existence must not deny this death which it carries in its heart; it must assert itself as an absolute in its very finiteness; man fulfills himself within the transitory or not at all. He must regard his undertakings as finite and will them absolutely.

It is obvious that this finiteness is not that of the pure instant; we have said that the future was the meaning and the substance of all action; the limits can not be marked out *a priori;* there are projects which define the future of a day or of an hour; and there are others which are inserted into structures capable of being developed through one, two, or several centuries, and thereby they have a concrete hold on one or two or several centuries. When one fights for the emancipation of oppressed natives, or the socialist revolution, he is obviously aiming at a long range goal; and he is still aiming at it concretely, beyond his own death, through the movement, the league, the institutions, or the party that he has helped set up. What we maintain is that one must not expect that this goal be justified as a point of departure of a new future; insofar as we no longer have a hold on the time which will flow beyond its coming, we must not expect anything of that time for which we have worked; other men will have to live its joys and sorrows. As for us, the goal must be considered as an end; we have to justify it on the basis of our freedom which has projected it, by the ensemble of the movement which ends in its fulfillment. The tasks we have set up for ourselves and which, though exceeding the limits of our lives, are ours, must find their meaning in themselves and not in a mythical Historical end.

But then, if we reject the idea of a future-myth in order to retain only that of a living and finite future, one which delimits transitory forms, we have not removed the antinomy of action; the present sacrifices and failures no longer seem compensated for in any point of time. And utility can no longer be defined absolutely. Thus, are we not ending by condemning action as criminal and absurd though at the same time condemning man to action?

Ambiguity

The notion of ambiguity must not be confused with that of absurdity. To declare that existence is absurd is to deny that it can ever be given a meaning; to say that it is ambiguous is to assert that its meaning is never fixed, that it must be constantly won. Absurdity challenges every ethics; but also the finished rationalization of the real would leave no room for ethics; it is because man's condition is ambiguous that he seeks, through failure and outrageousness, to save his existence. Thus, to say that action has to be lived in its truth, that is, in the consciousness of the antinomies which it involves, does not mean that one has to renounce it. In *Plutarch Lied* Pierrefeu rightly says that in war there is no victory which can not be regarded as unsuccessful, for the objective which one aims at is the total annihilation of the enemy and this result is never attained; yet there are wars which are won and wars which are lost. So is it with any activity; failure and success are two aspects of reality which at the start are not perceptible. That is what makes criticism so easy and art so difficult: the critic is always in a good position to show the limits that every artist gives himself in choosing himself; painting is not given completely either in Giotto or Titian or Cezanne; it is sought through the centuries and is never finished; a painting in which all pictorial problems are resolved is really inconceivable; painting itself is this movement toward its own reality; it is not the vain displacement of a millstone turning in the void; it concretizes itself on each canvas as an absolute existence. Art and science do not establish themselves despite failure but through it; which does not prevent there being truths and errors, masterpieces and lemons, depending upon whether the discovery or the painting has or has not known how to win the adherence of human consciousnesses; this amounts to saying that failure, always ineluctable, is in certain cases spared and in others not.

It is interesting to pursue this comparison; not that we are likening action to a work of art or a scientific theory, but because in any case human transcendence must cope with the same problem: it has to found itself, though it is prohibited from ever fulfilling itself. Now, we know that neither science nor art ever leaves it up to the future to justify its present existence. In no age does art consider itself as something which is paving the way for Art: so-called archaic art prepares for classicism only in the eyes of archaeologists; the sculptor who fashioned the Korai of Athens rightfully thought that he was producing a finished work of art; in no age has science considered itself as partial and lacunary;

without believing itself to be definitive, it has however, always wanted to be a total expression of the world, and it is in its totality that in each age it again raises the question of its own validity. There we have an example of how man must, in any event, assume his finiteness: not by treating his existence as transitory or relative but by reflecting the infinite within it, that is, by treating it as absolute. There is an art only because at every moment art has willed itself absolutely; likewise there is a liberation of man only if, in aiming at itself, freedom is achieved absolutely in the very fact of aiming at itself. This requires that each action be considered as a finished form whose different moments, instead of fleeing toward the future in order to find there their justification, reflect and confirm one another so well that there is no longer a sharp separation between present and future, between means and ends.

But if these moments constitute a unity, there must be no contradiction among them. Since the liberation aimed at is not a *thing* situated in an unfamiliar time, but a movement which realizes itself by tending to conquer, it can not attain itself if it denies itself at the start; action can not seek to fulfill itself by means which would destroy its very meaning. So much so that in certain situations there will be no other issue for man than rejection. In what is called political realism there is no room for rejection because the present is considered as transitory; there is rejection only if man lays claim in the present to his existence as an absolute value; then he must absolutely reject what would deny this value. Today, more or less consciously in the name of such an ethics, we condemn a magistrate who handed over a communist to save ten hostages and along with him all the Vichyites who were trying "to make the best of things:" it was not a matter of rationalizing the present such as it was imposed by the German occupation, but of rejecting it unconditionally. The resistance did not aspire to a positive effectiveness; it was a negation, a revolt, a martyrdom; and in this negative movement freedom was positively and absolutely confirmed.

In one sense the negative attitude is easy; the rejected object is given unequivocally and unequivocally defines the revolt that one opposes to it; thus, all French antifascists were united during the occupation by their common resistance to a single oppressor. The return to the positive encounters many more obstacles, as we have well seen in France where divisions and hatreds were revived at the same time as were the parties. In the moment of rejection, the antinomy of action is removed, and means and end meet; freedom immediately sets itself up as its own goal and fulfills itself by so doing. But the antinomy reappears as soon as freedom again gives itself ends which are far off in the future; then, through the resistances of the given, divergent means offer themselves and certain ones come to be seen as contrary to their ends. It has often been observed that revolt alone is pure. Every construction implies the outrage of dictatorship, of violence. This is the theme, among others, of Koestler's *Gladiators*. Those who, like this symbolic *Spartacus,* do not want to retreat from the outrage and resign themselves to impotence, usually seek refuge in the values of seriousness. That is why, among individuals as well as collectivities, the negative moment is often the most genuine. Goethe, Barres, and Aragon, disdainful or rebellious in their romantic youth, shattered old conformisms and thereby proposed a real, though incomplete, liberation. But what happened later on? Goethe became a servant of the state, Barres of nationalism, and Aragon of Stalinist conformism. We know how the seriousness of the Catholic Church was substituted for the Christian spirit, which was a rejection of dead Law, a subjective rapport of the individual with God through faith and charity; the Reformation was a revolt of subjectivity, but Protestantism in turn changed into an objective moralism in which the seriousness of works replaced the restlessness of faith. As for revolutionary humanism, it accepts only rarely the tension of permanent liberation; it has created a Church where salvation is bought by membership in a party as it is bought elsewhere by baptism and indulgences. We have seen that this recourse to the serious is a lie; it entails the sacrifice of man to the Thing, of freedom to the Cause. In order for the return to the positive to be genuine it must involve negativity, it must not conceal the antinomies between means and end, present and future; they must be lived in a permanent tension; one must retreat from neither the outrage of violence nor deny it, or, which amounts to the same thing, assume it lightly. Kierkegaard has said that what distinguishes the pharisee from the genuinely moral man is that the former considers his anguish as a sure sign of his virtue; from the fact that he asks himself, "Am I Abraham?" he concludes, "I am Abraham;" but morality resides in the painfulness of an indefinite questioning. The problem which we are posing is not the same as that of Kierkegaard; the important thing to us is to know whether, in given conditions, Isaac must be killed or not. But we also think that what distinguishes the tyrant from the man of good will is that the first rests in the certainty of his aims, whereas the second keeps asking himself, "Am I really working for the liberation of men? Isn't this end contested by the sacrifices through which I aim at it?" In setting up its ends, freedom must put them in parentheses, confront them at each moment with that absolute end which it itself constitutes, and contest, in its own name, the means it uses to win itself.

It will be said that these considerations remain quite abstract. What must be done, practically? Which action is good? Which is bad? To ask such a question is also to fall into a naive abstraction. We don't ask the physicist, "Which hypotheses are true?" Nor the artist, "By what procedures does one produce a work whose beauty is guaranteed?" Ethics does not furnish recipes any more than do science and art. One can merely propose methods. Thus, in science the fundamental problem is to make the idea adequate to its content and the law adequate to the facts; the logician finds that in the case where the pressure of the given fact bursts the concept which serves to comprehend it, one is obliged to invent another concept; but he can not define *a priori* the moment of invention, still less foresee it. Analogously, one may say that in the case where the content of the action falsifies its meaning, one must modify not the meaning, which is here willed absolutely, but the content itself; however, it is impossible to determine this relationship between meaning and content abstractly and universally: there must be a trial and decision in each case. But likewise just as the physicist finds it profitable to reflect on the conditions of scientific invention and the artist on those of artistic creation without expecting any ready-made solutions to come from these reflections, it is useful for the man of action to find out under what conditions his undertakings are valid. We are going to see that on this basis new perspectives are disclosed.

In the first place, it seems to us that the individual as such is one of the ends at which our action must aim. Here we are at one with the point of view of Christian charity, the Epicurean cult of friendship, and Kantian moralism which treats each man as an end. He interests us not merely as a member of a class, a nation, or a collectivity, but as an individual man. This distinguishes us from the systematic politician who cares only about collective destinies; and probably a tramp enjoying his bottle of wine, or a child playing with a balloon, or a Neapolitan lazzarone loafing in the sun in no way helps in the liberation of man; that is why the abstract will of the revolutionary scorns the concrete benevolence which occupies itself in satisfying desires which have no morrow. However, it must not be forgotten that there is a concrete bond between freedom and existence; to will man free is to will there to *be* being, it is to will the disclosure of being in the joy of existence; in order for the idea of liberation to have a concrete meaning, the joy of existence must be asserted in each one, at every instant; the movement toward freedom assumes its real, flesh and blood figure in the world by thickening into pleasure, into happiness. If the satisfaction of an old man drinking a glass of wine counts for nothing, then production and wealth are only hollow myths; they have meaning only if they are capable of being retrieved in individual and living joy. The saving of time and the conquest of leisure have no meaning if we are not moved by the laugh of a child at play. If we do not love life on our own account and through others, it is futile to seek to justify it in any way.

However, politics is right in rejecting benevolence to the extent that the latter thoughtlessly sacrifices the future to the present. The ambiguity of freedom, which very often is occupied only in fleeing from itself, introduces a difficult equivocation into relationships with each individual taken one by one. Just what is meant by the expression "to love others"? What is meant by taking them as ends? In any event, it is evident that we are not going to decide to fulfill the will of every man. There are cases where a man positively wants evil, that is, the enslavement of other men, and he must then be fought. It also happens that, without harming anyone, he flees from his own freedom, seeking passionately and alone to attain the being which constantly eludes him. If he asks for our help, are we to give it to him? We blame a man who helps a drug addict intoxicate himself or a desperate man commit suicide, for we think that rash behavior of this sort is an attempt of the individual against his own freedom; he must be made aware of his error and put in the presence of the real demands of his freedom. Well and good. But what if he persists? Must we then use violence? There again the serious man busies himself dodging the problem; the values of life, of health, and of moral conformism being set up, one does not hesitate to impose them on others. But we know that this pharisaism can cause the worst disasters: lacking drugs, the addict may kill himself. It is no more necessary to serve an abstract ethics obstinately than to yield without due consideration to impulses of pity or generosity; violence is justified only if it opens concrete possibilities to the freedom which I am trying to save; by practicing it I am willy-nilly assuming an engagement in relation to others and to myself; a man whom I snatch from the death which he had chosen has the right to come and ask me for means and reasons for living; the tyranny practiced against an invalid can be justified only by his getting better; whatever the purity of the intention which animates me, any dictatorship is a fault for which I have to get myself pardoned. Besides, I am in no position to make decisions of this sort indiscriminately; the example of the unknown person who throws himself in to the Seine and whom I hesitate whether or not to fish out is quite abstract; in the absence of a concrete bond with this desperate person my choice will never be anything but a contingent facticity. If I find myself in a position to do violence to a child, or to a melancholic, sick, or distraught person the reason is that I also find myself charged with his upbringing, his happiness, and his health: I am a parent, a teacher, a nurse, a doctor, or a friend... So, by a tacit agreement, by the very fact that I am solicited, the strictness of my decision is accepted or even desired; the more seriously I accept my responsibilities, the more justified it is. That is why love authorizes severities which are not granted to indifference. What makes the problem so complex is that, on the one hand, one must not make himself an accomplice of that flight from freedom that is found in heedlessness, caprice, mania, and passion, and that, on the other hand, it is the abortive movement of man toward being which is his very existence, it is through the failure which he has assumed that he asserts himself as a freedom. To want to prohibit a man from error is to forbid him to fulfill his own existence, it is to deprive him of life. At the beginning of Claudel's *The Satin Shoe,* the husband of Dona Prouheze, the judge, the just, as the author regards him, explains that every plant needs a gardener in order to grow and that he is the one whom heaven has destined for his young wife; beside the fact that we are shocked by the arrogance of such a thought (for how does he know that he is this enlightened gardener? Isn't he merely a jealous husband?) this likening of a soul to a plant is not acceptable; for, as Kant would say, the value of an act lies not in its *conformity* to an external model, but in its internal truth. We object to the inquisitors who want to create faith and virtue from without; we object to all forms of fascism which seek to fashion the happiness of man from without; and also the paternalism which thinks that it has done something for man by prohibiting him from certain possibilities of temptation, whereas what is necessary is to give him reasons for resisting it.

Thus, violence is not immediately justified when it opposes willful acts which one considers perverted; it becomes inadmissible if it uses the pretext of ignorance to deny a freedom which, as we have seen, can be practiced within ignorance itself. Let the "enlightened elites" strive to change the situation of the child, the illiterate, the primitive crushed beneath his superstitions; that is one of their most urgent tasks; but in this very effort they must respect a freedom which, like theirs, is absolute. They are always opposed, for example, to the extension of universal suffrage by adducing the incompetence of the masses, of women, of the natives in the colonies; but this forgetting that man always has to decide by himself in the darkness, that he must want beyond what he knows. If infinite knowledge were necessary (even supposing that it were conceivable), then the colonial administrator himself would not have the right to freedom; he is much further from perfect knowledge than the most backward savage is from him. Actually, to vote is not to govern; and to govern is not merely to maneuver; there is an ambiguity today, and particularly in France, because we think that we are not the master of our destiny; we no longer hope to help make history, we are resigned to submitting to it; all that our internal politics does is reflect the play of external forces, no party hopes to determine the fate of the country but merely to foresee the future which is being prepared in the world by foreign powers and to use, as best we can, the bit of indetermination which still escapes their foresight. Drawn along by this tactical realism, the citizens themselves no longer consider the vote as the assertion of their will but as a maneuver, whether one adheres completely to the maneuvering of a party or whether one invents his own strategy; the electors consider themselves not as men who are consulted about a particular point but as forces which are numbered and which are ordered about with a view to distant ends. And that is probably why the French, who formerly were so eager to declare their opinions, take no further interest in an act which has become a disheartening strategy. So, the fact is that if it is necessary not to vote but to measure the weight of one's vote, this calculation requires such extensive information and such a sureness of foresight that only a specialized technician can have the boldness to express an opinion. But that is one of the abuses whereby the whole meaning of democracy is lost; the logical conclusion of this would be to suppress the vote. The vote should really be the expression of a concrete will, the choice of a representative capable of defending, within the general framework of the country and the world, the particular interests of his electors. The ignorant and the outcast also has interests to defend; he alone is "competent" to decide upon his hopes and his trust. By a sophism which leans upon the dishonesty of the serious, one does not merely argue about his formal impotence to choose, but one draws arguments from the content of his choice. I recall, among others, the naivete of a right-thinking young girl who said, "The vote for women is all well and good in principle, only, if women get the vote, they'll all vote red." With like impudence it is almost unanimously stated today in France that if the natives of the French Union were given the rights of self-determination, they would live quietly in their villages without doing anything, which would be harmful to the higher interests of the Economy.

And doubtless the state of stagnation in which they choose to live is not that which a man can wish for another man; it is desirable to open new possibilities to the indolent negroes so that the interests of the Economy may one day merge with theirs. But for the time being, they are left to vegetate in the sort of situation where their freedom can merely be negative – the best thing they can desire is not to tire themselves, not to suffer, and not to work; and even this freedom is denied them. It is the most consummate and inacceptable form of oppression.

However, the "enlightened elite" objects, one does not let a child dispose of himself, one does not permit him to vote. This is another sophism. To the extent that woman or the happy or resigned slave lives in the infantile world of ready-made values, calling them "an eternal child" or a "grown-up child" has some meaning, but the analogy is only partial. Childhood is a particular sort of situation: it is a natural situation whose limits are not created by other men and which is thereby not comparable to a situation of oppression; it is a situation which is common to all men and which is temporary for all; therefore, it does not represent a limit which cuts off the individual from his possibilities, but, on the contrary, the moment of a development in which new possibilities are won. The child is ignorant because he has not yet had the time to acquire knowledge, not because this time has been refused him. To treat him as a child is not to bar him from the future but to open it to him; he needs to be taken in hand, he invites authority, it is the form which the resistance of facticity, through which all liberation is brought about, takes for him. And on the other hand, even in this situation the child has a right to his freedom and must be respected as a human person. What gives *Emile* its value is the brilliance with which Rousseau asserts this principle. There is a very annoying naturalistic optimism in *Emile;* in the rearing of the child, as in any relationship with others, the ambiguity of freedom implies the outrage of violence; in a sense, all education is a failure. But Rousseau is right in refusing to allow childhood to be oppressed. And in practice raising a child as one cultivates a plant which one does not consult about its needs is very different from considering it as a freedom to whom the future must be opened.

Thus, we can set up point number one: the good of an individual or a group of individuals requires that it be taken as an absolute end of our action; but we are not authorized to decide upon this end *a priori.* The fact is that no behavior is ever authorized to begin with, and one of the concrete consequences of existentialist ethics is the rejection of all the previous justifications which might be drawn from the civilization, the age, and the culture; it is the rejection of every principle of authority. To put it positively, the precept will be to treat the other (to the extent that he is the only one concerned, which is the moment that we are considering at present) as a freedom so that his end may be freedom; in using this conducting wire one will have to incur the risk, in each case, of inventing an original solution. Out of disappointment in love a young girl takes an overdose of phenolbarbital; in the morning friends find her dying, they call a doctor, she is saved; later on she becomes a happy mother of a family; her friends were right in considering her suicide as a hasty and heedless act and in putting her into a position to reject it or return to it freely. But in asylums one sees melancholic patients who have tried to commit suicide twenty times, who devote their freedom to seeking the means of escaping their jailers and of putting an end to their intolerable anguish; the doctor who gives them a friendly pat on the shoulder is their tyrant and their torturer. A friend who is intoxicated by alcohol or drugs asks me for money so that he can go and buy the poison that is necessary to him; I urge him to get cured, I take him to a doctor, I try to help him live; insofar as there is a chance of my being successful, I am acting correctly in refusing him the sum he asks for. But if circumstances prohibit me from doing anything to change the situation in which he is struggling, all I can do is give in; a deprivation of a few hours will do nothing but exasperate his torments uselessly; and he may have recourse to extreme means to get what I do not give him. That is also the problem touched on by Ibsen in *The Wild Duck*. An individual lives in a situation of falsehood; the falsehood is violence, tyranny: shall I tell the truth in order to free the victim? It would first be necessary to create a situation of such a kind that the truth might be bearable and that, though losing his illusions, the deluded individual might again find about him reasons for hoping. What makes the problem more complex is that the freedom of one man almost always concerns that of other individuals. Here is a married couple who persist in living in a hovel; if one does not succeed in giving them the desire to live in a more healthful dwelling, they must be allowed to follow their preferences; but the situation changes if they have children; the freedom of the parents would be the ruin of their sons, and as freedom and the future are on the side of the latter, these are the ones who must first be taken into account. The Other is multiple, and on the basis of this new questions arise.

One might first wonder for whom we are seeking freedom and happiness. When raised in this way, the problem is abstract; the answer will, therefore, be arbitrary, and the arbitrary always involves outrage. It is not entirely the fault of the district social-worker if she is apt to be odious; because, her money and time being limited, she hesitates before distributing it to this one or that one, she appears to others as a pure externality, a blind facticity. Contrary to the formal strictness of Kantianism for whom the more abstract the act is the more virtuous it is, generosity seems to us to be better grounded and therefore more valid the less distinction there is between the other and ourself and the more we fulfill ourself in taking the other as an end. That is what happens if I am engaged in relation to others. The Stoics impugned the ties of family, friendship, and nationality so that they recognized only the universal form of man. But man is man only through situations whose particularity is precisely a universal fact. There are men who expect help from certain men and not from others, and these expectations define privileged lines of action. It is fitting that the negro fight for the negro, the Jew for the Jew, the proletarian for the proletarian, and the Spaniard in Spain. But the assertion of these particular solidarities must not contradict the will for universal solidarity and each finite undertaking must also be open on the totality of men.

But it is then that we find in concrete form the conflicts which we have described abstractly; for the cause of freedom can triumph only through particular sacrifices. And certainly there are hierarchies among the goods desired by men: one will not hesitate to sacrifice the comfort, luxury, and leisure of certain men to assure the liberation of certain others; but when it is a question of choosing among freedoms, how shall we decide?

Let us repeat, one can only indicate a method here. The first point is always to consider what genuine human interest fills the abstract form which one proposes as the action's end. Politics always puts forward Ideas: Nation, Empire, Union, Economy, etc. But none of these forms has value in itself; it has it only insofar as it involves concrete individuals. If a nation can assert itself proudly only to the detriment of its members, if a union can be created only to the detriment of those it is trying to unite, the nation or the union must be rejected. We repudiate all idealisms, mysticisms, etcetera which prefer a Form to man himself. But the matter becomes really agonizing when it is a question of a Cause which genuinely serves man. That is why the question of Stalinist politics, the problem of the relationship of the Party to the masses which it uses in order to serve them, is in the forefront of the preoccupations of all men of good will. However, there are very few who raise it without dishonesty, and we must first try to dispel a few fallacies.

The opponent of the U.S.S.R. is making use of a fallacy when, emphasizing the part of criminal violence assumed by Stalinist politics, he neglects to confront it with the ends pursued. Doubtless, the purges, the deportations, the abuses of the occupation, and the police dictatorship surpass in importance the violences practiced by any other country; the very fact that there are a hundred and sixty million inhabitants in Russia multiplies the numerical coefficient of the injustices committed. But these quantitative considerations are insufficient. One can no more judge the means without the end which gives it its meaning than he can detach the end from the means which defines it. Lynching a negro or suppressing a hundred members of the opposition are two analogous acts. Lynching is an absolute evil; it represents the survival of an obsolete civilization, the perpetuation of a struggle of races which has to disappear; it is a fault without justification or excuse. Suppressing a hundred opponents is surely an outrage, but it may have meaning and a reason; it is a matter of maintaining a regime which brings to an immense mass of men a bettering of their lot. Perhaps this measure could have been avoided; perhaps it merely represents that necessary element of failure which is involved in any positive construction. It can be judged only by being replaced in the ensemble of the cause it serves.

But, on the other hand, the defender of the U.S.S.R. is making use of a fallacy when he unconditionally justifies the sacrifices and the crimes by the ends pursued; it would first be necessary to prove that, on the one hand, the end is unconditioned and that, on the other hand, the crimes committed in its name were strictly necessary. Against the death of Bukharin one counters with Stalingrad; but one would have to know to what effective extent the Moscow trials increased the chances of the Russian victory. One of the ruses of Stalinist orthodoxy is, playing on the idea of necessity, to put the whole of the revolution on one side of the scale; the other side will always seem very light. But the very idea of a total dialectic of history does not imply that any factor is ever determining; on the contrary, if one admits that the life of a man may change the course of events, it is that one adheres to the conception which grants a preponderant role to Cleopatra's nose and Cromwell's wart. One is here playing, with utter dishonesty, on two opposite conceptions of the idea of necessity: one synthetic, and the other analytic; one dialectic, the other deterministic. The first makes History appear as an intelligible becoming within which the particularity of contingent accidents is reabsorbed; the dialectical sequence of the moments is possible only if there is within each moment an indetermination of the particular elements taken one by one. If, on the contrary, one grants the strict determinism of each causal series, one ends in a contingent and disordered vision of the ensemble, the conjunction of the series being brought about by chance. Therefore, a Marxist must recognize that none of his particular decisions involves the revolution in its totality; it is merely a matter of hastening or retarding its coming, of saving himself the use of other and more costly means. That does not mean that he must retreat from violence but that he must not regard it as justified *a priori* by its ends. If he considers his enterprise in its truth, that is, in its finiteness, he will understand that he has never anything but a finite stake to oppose to the sacrifices which he calls for, and that it is an uncertain stake. Of course, this uncertainty should not keep him from pursuing his goals; but it requires that one concern himself in each case with finding a balance between the goal and its means.

Thus, we challenge every condemnation as well as every *a priori* justification of the violence practiced with a view to a valid end. They must be legitimized concretely. A calm, mathematical calculation is here impossible. One must attempt to judge the chances of success that are involved in a certain sacrifice; but at the beginning this judgment will always be doubtful; besides, in the face of the immediate reality of the sacrifice, the notion of chance is difficult to think about. On the one hand, one can multiply a probability infinitely without ever reaching certainty; but yet, practically, it ends by merging with this asymptote: in our private life as in our collective life there is no other truth than a statistical one. On the other hand, the interests at stake do not allow themselves to be put into an equation; the suffering of one man, that of a million men, are incommensurable with the conquests realized by millions of others, present death is incommensurable with the life to come. It would be utopian to want to set up on the one hand the chances of success multiplied by the stake one is after, and on the other hand the weight of the immediate sacrifice. One finds himself back at the anguish of free decision. And that is why political choice is an ethical choice: it is a wager as well as a decision; one bets on the chances and risks of the measure under consideration; but whether chances and risks must be assumed or not in the given circumstances must be decided without help, and in so doing one sets up values. If in 1793 the Girondists rejected the violences of the Terror whereas a Saint-Just and a Robespierre assumed them, the reason is that they did not have the same conception of freedom. Nor was the same republic being aimed at between 1830 and 1840 by the republicans who limited themselves to a purely political opposition and those who adopted the technique of insurrection. In each case it is a matter of defining an end and realizing it, knowing that the choice of the means employed affects both the definition and the fulfillment.

Ordinarily, situations are so complex that a long analysis is necessary before being able to pose the ethical moment of the choice. We shall confine ourselves here to the consideration of a few simple examples which will enable us to make our attitude somewhat more precise. In an underground revolutionary movement when one discovers the presence of a stool-pigeon, one does not hesitate to beat him up; he is a present and future danger who has to be gotten rid of; but if a man is merely suspected of treason, the case is more ambiguous. We blame those northern peasants who in the war of 1914-18 massacred an innocent family which was suspected of signaling to the enemy; the reason is that not only were the presumptions vague, but the danger was uncertain; at any rate, it was enough to put the suspects into prison; while waiting for a serious inquiry it was easy to keep them from doing any harm. However, if a questionable individual holds the fate of other men in his hands, if, in order to avoid the risk of killing one innocent man, one runs the risk of letting ten innocent men die, it is reasonable to sacrifice him. We can merely ask that such decisions be not taken hastily and lightly, and that, all things considered, the evil that one inflicts be lesser than that which is being forestalled.

There are cases still more disturbing because there the violence is not immediately efficacious; the violences of the Resistance did not aim at the material weakening of Germany; it happens that their purpose was to create such a state of violence that collaboration would be impossible; in one sense, the burning of a whole French village was too high a price to pay for the elimination of three enemy officers; but those fires and the massacring of hostages were themselves parts of the plan; they created an abyss between the occupiers and the occupied. Likewise, the insurrections in Paris and Lyons at the beginning of the nineteenth century, or the revolts in India, did not aim at shattering the yoke of the oppressor at one blow, but rather at creating and keeping alive the meaning of the revolt and at making the mystifications of conciliation impossible. Attempts which are aware that one by one they are doomed to failure can be legitimized by the whole of the situation which they create. This is also the meaning of Steinbeck's novel *In Dubious Battle* where a communist leader does not hesitate to launch a costly strike of uncertain success but through which there will be born, along with the solidarity of the workers, the consciousness of exploitation and the will to reject it.

It seems to me interesting to contrast this example with the debate in John Dos Passos' *The Adventures of a Young Man.* Following a strike, some American miners are condemned to death. Their comrades try to have their trial reconsidered. Two methods are put forward: one can act officially, and one knows that they then have an excellent chance of winning their case; one can also work up a sensational trial with the Communist Party taking the affair in hand, stirring up a press campaign and circulating international petitions; but the court will be unwilling to yield to this intimidation. The party will thereby get a tremendous amount of publicity, but the miners will be condemned. What is a man of good will to decide in this case? Dos Passos' hero chooses to save the miners and we believe that he did right. Certainly, if it were necessary to choose between the whole revolution and the lives of two or three men, no revolutionary would hesitate; but it was merely a matter of helping along the party propaganda, or better, of increasing somewhat its chances of developing within the United States; the immediate interest of the C.P. in that country is only hypothetically tied up with that of the revolution; in fact, a cataclysm like the war has so upset the situation of the world that a great part of the gains and losses of the past have been absolutely swept away. If it is really men which the movement claims to be serving, in this case it must prefer saving the lives of three concrete individuals to a very uncertain and weak chance of serving a little more effectively by their sacrifice the mankind to come. If it considers these lives negligible, it is because it too ranges itself on the side of the formal politicians who prefer the Idea to its content; it is because it prefers itself, in its subjectivity, to the goals to which it claims to be dedicated. Besides, whereas in the example chosen by Steinbeck the strike is immediately an appeal to the freedom of the workers and in its very failure is already a liberation, the sacrifice of the miners is a mystification and an oppression; they are duped by being made to believe that an effort is being made to save their lives, and the whole proletariat is duped with them. Thus, in both examples, we find ourselves before the same abstract case: men are going to die so that the party which claims to be serving them will realize a limited gain; but a concrete analysis leads us to opposite moral solutions.

It is apparent that the method we are proposing, analogous in this respect to scientific or aesthetic methods, consists, in each case, of confronting the values realized with the values aimed at, and the meaning of the act with its content. The fact is that the politician, contrary to the scientist and the artist, and although the element of failure which he assumes is much more outrageous, is rarely concerned with making use of it. May it be that there is an irresistible dialectic of power wherein morality has no place? Is the ethical concern, even in its realistic and concrete form, detrimental to the interests of action? The objection will surely be made that hesitation and misgivings only impede victory. Since, in any case, there is an element of failure in all success, since the ambiguity, at any rate, must be surmounted, why not refuse to take notice of it? In the first number of the *Cahiers d'Action* a reader declared that once and for all we should regard the militant communist as "the permanent hero of our time" and should reject the exhausting tension demanded by existentialism; installed in the permanence of heroism, he will blindly direct himself toward an uncontested goal; but one then resembles Colonel de la Roque who unwaveringly went right straight ahead of him without knowing where he was going. Malaparte relates that the young Nazis, in order to become insensitive to the suffering of others, practiced by plucking out the eyes of live cats; there is no more radical way of avoiding the pitfalls of ambiguity. But an action which wants to serve man ought to be careful not to forget him on the way; if it chooses to fulfill itself blindly, it will lose its meaning or will take on an unforeseen meaning; for the goal is not fixed once and for all; it is defined all along the road which leads to it. Vigilance alone can keep alive the validity of the goals and the genuine assertion of freedom. Moreover, ambiguity can not fail to appear on the scene; it is felt by the victim, and his revolt or his complaints also make it exist for his tyrant; the latter will then be tempted to put everything into question, to renounce, thus denying both himself and his ends; or, if he persists, he will continue to blind himself only by multiplying crimes and by perverting his original design more and more. The fact is that the man of action becomes a dictator not in respect to his ends but because these ends are necessarily set up through his will. Hegel, in his *Phenomenology,* has emphasized this inextricable confusion between objectivity and subjectivity. A man gives himself to a Cause only by making it *his* Cause; as he fulfills himself within it, it is also through him that it is expressed, and the will to power is not distinguished in such a case from generosity; when an individual or a party chooses to triumph, whatever the cost may be, it is their own triumph which they take for an end. If the fusion of the Commissar and the Yogi were realized, there would be a self-criticism in the man of action which would expose to him the ambiguity of his will, thus arresting the imperious drive of his subjectivity and, by the same token, contesting the unconditioned value of the goal. But the fact is that the politician follows the line of least resistance; it is easy to fall asleep over the unhappiness of others and to count it for very little; it is easier to throw a hundred men, ninety-seven of whom are innocent, into prison, than to discover the three culprits who are hidden among them; it is easier to kill a man than to keep a close watch on him; all politics makes use of the police, which officially flaunts its radical contempt for the individual and which loves violence for its own sake. The thing that goes by the name of political necessity is in part the laziness and brutality of the police. That is why it is incumbent upon ethics not to follow the line of least resistance; an act which is not destined, but rather quite freely consented to; it must make itself effective so that what was at first facility may become difficult. For want of internal criticism, this is the role that an opposition must take upon itself. There are two types of opposition. The first is a rejection of the very ends set up by a regime: it is the opposition of anti-fascism to fascism, of fascism to socialism. In the second type, the oppositionist accepts the objective goal but criticizes the subjective movement which aims at it; he may not even wish for a change of power, but he deems it necessary to bring into play a contestation which will make the subjective appear as such. Thereby he exacts a perpetual contestation of the means by the end and of the end by the means. He must be careful himself not to ruin, by the means which he employs, the end he is aiming at, and above all not to pass into the service of the oppositionists of the first type. But, delicate as it may be, his role is, nevertheless, necessary. Indeed, on the one hand, it would be absurd to oppose a liberating action with the pretext that it implies crime and tyranny; for without crime and tyranny there could be no liberation of man; one can not escape that dialectic which goes from freedom to freedom through dictatorship and oppression. But, on the other hand, he would be guilty of allowing the liberating movement to harden into a moment which is acceptable only if it passes into its opposite; tyranny and crime must be kept from triumphantly establishing themselves in the world; the conquest of freedom is their only justification, and the assertion of freedom against them must therefore be kept alive.

Conclusion

Is this kind of ethics individualistic or not? Yes, if one means by that that it accords to the individual an absolute value and that it recognizes in him alone the power of laying the foundations of his own existence. It is individualism in the sense in which the wisdom of the ancients, the Christian ethics of salvation, and the Kantian ideal of virtue also merit this name; it is opposed to the totalitarian doctrines which raise up beyond man the mirage of Mankind. But it is not solipsistic, since the individual is defined only by his relationship to the world and to other individuals; he exists only by transcending himself, and his freedom can be achieved only through the freedom of others. He justifies his existence by a movement which, like freedom, springs from his heart but which leads outside of him.

This individualism does not lead to the anarchy of personal whim. Man is free; but he finds his law in his very freedom. First, he must assume his freedom and not flee it by a constructive movement: one does not exist without doing something; and also by a negative movement which rejects oppression for oneself and others. In construction, as in rejection, it is a matter of reconquering freedom on the contingent facticity of existence, that is, of taking the given, which, at the start, *is there* without any reason, as something willed by man.

A conquest of this kind is never finished; the contingency remains, and, so that he may assert his will, man is even obliged to stir up in the world the outrage he does not want. But this element of failure is a very condition of his life; one can never dream of eliminating it without immediately dreaming of death. This does not mean that one should consent to failure, but rather one must consent to struggle against it without respite.

Yet, isn't this battle without victory pure gullibility? It will be argued that this is only a ruse of transcendence projecting before itself a goal which constantly recedes, running after itself on an endless treadmill; to exist for Mankind is to remain where one is, and it fools itself by calling this turbulent stagnation progress; our whole ethics does nothing but encourage it in this lying enterprise since we are asking each one to confirm existence as a value for all others; isn't it simply a matter of organizing among men a complicity which allows them to substitute a game of illusions for the given world?

We have already attempted to answer this objection. One can formulate it only by placing himself on the grounds of an inhuman and consequently false objectivity; within Mankind men may be fooled; the word "lie" has a meaning by opposition to the truth established by men themselves, but Mankind can not fool itself completely since it is precisely Mankind which creates the criteria of true and false. In Plato, art is mystification because there is the heaven of Ideas; but in the earthly domain all glorification of the earth is true as soon as it is realized. Let men attach value to words, forms, colors, mathematical theorems, physical laws, and athletic prowess; let them accord value to one another in love and friendship, and the objects, the events, and the men immediately *have* this value; they have it absolutely. It is possible that a man may refuse to love anything on earth; he will prove this refusal and he will carry it out by suicide. If he lives, the reason is that, whatever he may say, there still remains in him some attachment to existence; his life will be commensurate with this attachment; it will justify itself to the extent that it genuinely justifies the world.

This justification, though open upon the entire universe through time and space, will always be finite. Whatever one may do, one never realizes anything but a limited work, like existence itself which tries to establish itself through that work and which death also limits. It is the assertion of our finiteness which doubtless gives the doctrine which we have just evoked its austerity and, in some eyes, its sadness. As soon as one considers a system abstractly and theoretically, one puts himself, in effect, on the plane of the universal, thus, of the infinite. That is why reading the Hegelian system is so comforting. I remember having experienced a great feeling of calm on reading Hegel in the impersonal framework of the Bibliotheque Nationale in August 1940. But once I got into the street again, into my life, out of the system, beneath a real sky, the system was no longer of any use to me: what it had offered me, under a show of the infinite, was the consolations of death; and I again wanted to live in the midst of living men. I think that, inversely, existentialism does not offer to the reader the consolations of an abstract evasion: existentialism proposes no evasion. On the contrary, its ethics is experienced in the truth of life, and it then appears as the only proposition of salvation which one can address to men. Taking on its own account Descartes' revolt against the evil genius, the pride of the thinking reed in the face of the universe which crushes him, it asserts that, despite his limits, through them, it is up to each one to fulfill his existence as an absolute. Regardless of the staggering dimensions of the world about us, the density of our ignorance, the risks of catastrophes to come, and our individual weakness within the immense collectivity, the fact remains that we are absolutely free today if we choose to will our existence in its finiteness, a finiteness which is open on the infinite. And in fact, any man who has known real loves, real revolts, real desires, and real will knows quite well that he has no need of any outside guarantee to be sure of his goals; their certitude comes from his own drive. There is a very old saying which goes: "Do what you must, come what may." That amounts to saying in a different way that the result is not external to the good will which fulfills itself in aiming at it. If it came to be that each man did what he must, existence would be saved in each one without there being any need of dreaming of a paradise where all would be reconciled in death.

The End.

Biography

Simone De Beauvoir, (1908-1986)

French writer and <u>feminist</u>, and <u>Existentialist</u>. She is known primarily for her treatise <u>The Second Sex</u> (1949), a scholarly and passionate plea for the abolition of what she called the myth of the "eternal feminine." It became a classic of feminist literature during the 1960s.

Schooled in private institutions, de Beauvoir attended the Sorbonne, where, in 1929, she passed her agrégation in philosophy and met <u>Jean-Paul Sartre</u>, beginning a free, lifelong association with him. She taught at a number of schools (1931-43) before turning to writing for her livelihood. In 1945 she began editing *Le Temps Modernes* with Sartre.

Her novels expounded the major Existential themes, demonstrating her conception of the writer's commitment to the times. She Came To Stay (1943) treats the difficult problem of the relationship of a conscience to "<u>the other</u>". Of her other works of fiction, perhaps the best known is The Mandarins (1954), a chronicle of the attempts of post-World War II intellectuals to leave their "mandarin" (educated elite) status and engage in political activism. She also wrote four books of philosophy, including <u>The Ethics of Ambiguity</u> (1947).

Several volumes of her work are devoted to autobiography which constitute a telling portrait of French intellectual life from the 1930s to the 1970s. In addition to treating feminist issues, de Beauvoir was concerned with the issue of aging, which she addressed in A Very Easy Death (1964), on her mother's death in a hospital. In 1981 she wrote A Farewell to Sartre, a painful account of Sartre's last years.

Simone de Beauvoir revealed herself as a woman of formidable courage and integrity, whose life supported her thesis: the basic options of an individual must be made on the premises of an equal vocation for man and woman founded on a common structure of their being, independent of their sexuality.

CPSIA information can be obtained
at www.ICGtesting.com
Printed in the USA
BVHW011101080819
555409BV00005B/660/P

9 781461 134886